WG 140 Hou

MAKING SENSE OF THE ECG

MAKING SENSE OF THE ECG

A HANDS-ON GUIDE

Second Edition

Andrew R. Houghton

MA(Oxon.), DM, BM BCh, MRCP(UK)
Consultant Cardiologist,
Grantham & District Hospital,
Grantham, Lincolnshire, UK
and
Visiting Cardiologist,
Glenfield Hospital,
Leicester, UK

David Gray

DM, MPH, BMedSci, BM BS, FRCP(UK), FRIPH
Reader in Medicine and Honorary Consultant Physician,
Department of Cardiovascular Medicine,
University Hospital, Queen's Medical Centre, Nottingham, UK

A member of the Hodder Headline Group
LONDON

First published in Great Britain in 2003 by
Arnold, a member of the Hodder Headline Group,
338 Euston Road, London NW1 3BH

http://www.arnoldpublishers.com

Distributed in the United States of America by
Oxford University Press Inc.,
198 Madison Avenue, New York, NY 10016
Oxford is a registered trademark of Oxford University Press

Whilst the advice and information in this book are believed to be true and accurate
at the date of going to press, neither the authors nor the publisher can accept any
legal responsibility or liability for any errors or omissions that may be made. In
particular (but without limiting the generality of the preceding disclaimer) every
effort has been made to check drug dosages; however, it is still possible that errors
have been missed. Furthermore, dosage schedules are constantly being revised and
new side-effects recognized. For these reasons the reader is strongly urged to
consult the drug companies' printed instructions before administering any of the
drugs recommended in this book.

British Library Cataloguing in Publication Data
A catalogue record for this book is available from the British Library

Library of Congress Cataloging-in-Publication Data
A catalog record for this book is available from the Library of Congress

ISBN 0 340 80978 7
ISBN 0 340 81142 0 (International Students' Edition – restricted
territorial availability)

3 4 5 6 7 8 9 10

Commissioning Editor: Georgina Bentliff
Development Editor: Heather Smith
Project Editor: Wendy Rooke
Production Controller: Lindsay Smith
Cover Design: Amina Dudhia

Typeset in 10.5/13 Rotis Serif by Charon Tec Pvt. Ltd, Chennai, India
Printed and bound in Italy by Printer Trento S.r.l.

What do you think about this book? Or any other Arnold title?
Please send your comments to feedback.arnold@hodder.co.uk

To Kathryn & Caroline

CONTENTS

WHERE TO FIND
THE ECGs

WHERE TO FIND THE MEDICAL CONDITIONS

PREFACE TO THE SECOND EDITION

The first edition of *Making Sense of the ECG: A hands-on guide* proved to be a great success: it was awarded the prestigious Sir Richard Asher Prize of the Society of Medical Authors for 'Best First Textbook' in 1997; it received a Commendation in the British Medical Association Book Competition in 1998; and it was translated into ten languages.

Producing a second edition was quite a challenge for us to retain the style, layout, accessibility and spirit of the first edition while adding new sections and updating others.

Electrocardiographs have been replaced where we have been fortunate to acquire better examples. Information on new diagnostic markers of myocyte necrosis and on 'acute coronary syndromes' has been added. The section on cardiopulmonary resuscitation has been revised in accordance with the latest European Society of Cardiology/American College of Cardiology guidelines. The chapter on pacemakers has been expanded to cover automatic implantable cardioverter defibrillators. There is a new section on ambulatory ECG monitoring in the investigation of palpitations and suspected abnormal cardiac rhythms; readers who wish to know more about the aetiology and management of arrhythmias should consult David Bennett's excellent book *Cardiac Arrhythmias*.

Once again, we are grateful to all the staff at Hodder Arnold who have contributed to the success of *Making Sense of the ECG: A hands-on guide.*

Andrew Houghton
David Gray
April 2003

ACKNOWLEDGEMENTS

We would like to thank everyone who gave us suggestions and constructive criticism while we prepared the first and second editions of *Making Sense of the ECG*. We are particularly grateful to the following for their invaluable comments on the text and for allowing us to use ECGs from their collections:

Khin Maung Aye	Yuji Murakawa
Gabriella Captur	Francis Murgatroyd
Ian Ferrer	V.B.S. Naidu
Michael Holmes	George B. Pradhān
Safiy Karim	Catherine Scott
Dave Kendall	Neville Smith
Iain Lyburn	Gary Spiers
Sonia Lyburn	Andrew Stein
Martin Melville	Upul Wijayawardhana

We would also like to express our gratitude to everyone at Hodder Arnold for their guidance and support.

1

PQRST: WHERE THE WAVES COME FROM

The electrocardiogram (ECG) is one of the most widely used and useful investigations in contemporary medicine. It is essential for the identification of disorders of the cardiac rhythm, extremely useful for the diagnosis of abnormalities of the heart (such as myocardial infarction), and a helpful clue to the presence of generalized disorders that affect the rest of the body too (such as electrolyte disturbances).

Each chapter in this book considers a specific feature of the ECG in turn. We begin, however, with an overview of the ECG in which we explain the following points:

- What does the ECG actually record?
- How does the ECG 'look' at the heart?
- Where do the waves come from?
- How do I record an ECG?

We recommend you take some time to read through this chapter before trying to interpret ECG abnormalities.

WHAT DOES THE ECG ACTUALLY RECORD?

ECG machines record the electrical activity of the heart. They also pick up the activity of other muscles, such as skeletal muscle, but are designed to filter this out as much as possible.

Encouraging patients to relax during an ECG recording helps to obtain a clear trace (Fig. 1.1).

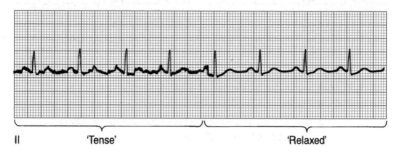

Fig. 1.1 An ECG from a relaxed patient is much easier to interpret

Key points: ● electrical interference (irregular baseline) when patient is tense
● clearer recording when patient relaxes

By convention, the main waves on the ECG are given the names P, Q, R, S, T and U (Fig. 1.2). Each wave represents depolarization ('electrical discharging') or repolarization ('electrical recharging') of a certain region of the heart – this is discussed in more detail in the rest of this chapter.

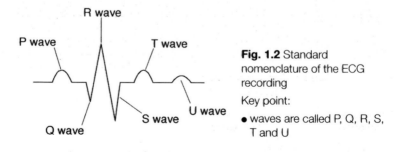

Fig. 1.2 Standard nomenclature of the ECG recording

Key point:
● waves are called P, Q, R, S, T and U

The voltage changes detected by ECG machines are very small, being of the order of millivolts. The size of each wave corresponds to the amount of voltage generated by the event that created it: the greater the voltage, the larger the wave (Fig. 1.3).

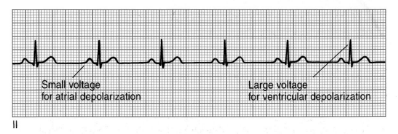

II

Fig. 1.3 The size of a wave reflects the voltage that caused it

Key points: • P waves are small (atrial depolarization generates little voltage)

• QRS complexes are larger (ventricular depolarization generates a higher voltage)

The ECG also allows you to calculate how long an event lasted. The ECG paper moves through the machine at a constant rate of 25 mm/s, so by measuring the width of a P wave, for example, you can calculate the duration of atrial depolarization (Fig. 1.4).

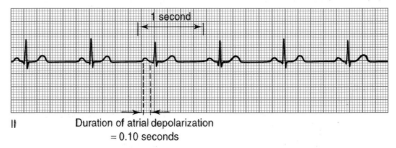

II   Duration of atrial depolarization
                    = 0.10 seconds

1 large square =   1 small square =
0.2 seconds   0.04 seconds

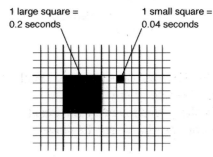

Fig. 1.4 The width of a wave reflects an event's duration

Key points:

• the P waves are 2.5 mm wide

• atrial depolarization therefore took 0.10 s

HOW DOES THE ECG 'LOOK' AT THE HEART?

To make sense of the ECG, one of the most important concepts to understand is that of the 'lead'. This is a term you will often see, and it does *not* refer to the wires that connect the patient to the ECG machine (which we will always refer to as 'electrodes' to avoid confusion).

In short, 'leads' are different viewpoints of the heart's electrical activity. An ECG machine uses the information it collects via its four limb and six chest electrodes to compile a comprehensive picture of the electrical activity in the heart as observed from 12 different viewpoints, and this set of 12 views or leads gives the 12-lead ECG its name.

Each lead is given a name (I, II, III, aVR, aVL, aVF, V_1, V_2, V_3, V_4, V_5 and V_6) and its position on a 12-lead ECG is usually standardized to make pattern recognition easier.

So what viewpoint does each lead have of the heart? Information from the four limb electrodes is used by the ECG machine to create the six limb leads (I, II, III, aVR, aVL and aVF). Each limb lead 'looks' at the heart from the side (the coronal plane), and the angle at which it looks at the heart in this plane depends upon the lead in question (Fig. 1.5). Thus, lead aVR looks at the heart from the approximate viewpoint of the patient's right shoulder, whereas lead aVL looks from the left shoulder and lead aVF looks directly upward from the feet.

The six chest leads (V_1 to V_6) look at the heart in a horizontal plane from the front and around the side of the chest (Fig. 1.6).

The region of myocardium surveyed by each lead therefore varies according to its vantage point – lead aVF has a good 'view' of the inferior surface of the heart, and lead V_3 has a good view of the anterior surface, for example.

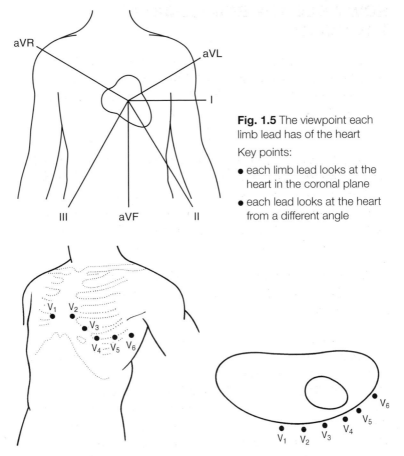

Fig. 1.5 The viewpoint each limb lead has of the heart

Key points:

- each limb lead looks at the heart in the coronal plane
- each lead looks at the heart from a different angle

Fig. 1.6 The viewpoint each chest lead has of the heart

Key points:
- each chest lead looks at the heart in the transverse plane
- each lead looks at the heart from a different angle

Once you know the view each lead has of the heart, you can tell if the electrical impulses in the heart are flowing towards that lead or away from it. This is very simple to work out, because electrical current flowing towards a lead produces an upward (positive) deflection on the ECG, whereas current flowing away causes a downward (negative) deflection (Fig. 1.7).

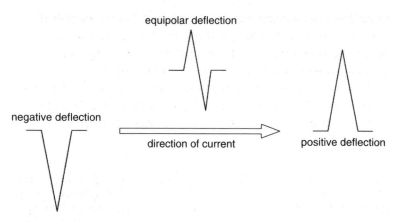

equipolar deflection

negative deflection

direction of current

positive deflection

Fig. 1.7 The direction of an ECG deflection depends upon the direction of the current

Key points:
- flow towards a lead produces a positive deflection
- flow away from a lead produces a negative deflection
- flow past a lead produces a positive then a negative (equipolar) deflection

We will discuss the origin of each wave shortly, but just as an example consider the P wave, which represents atrial depolarization. The P wave is positive in lead II because atrial depolarization flows towards that lead, but it is negative in lead aVR because this lead looks at the atria from the opposite direction (Fig. 1.8).

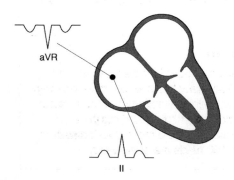

aVR

II

Fig. 1.8 The orientation of the P wave depends upon the lead

Key points:
- P waves are normally upright in lead II
- P waves are normally inverted in lead aVR

In addition to working out the direction of flow of electrical current, knowing the viewpoint of each lead allows you to determine which regions of the heart are affected by, for example, a myocardial infarction. Infarction of the inferior surface will produce changes in the leads looking at that region, namely leads II, III and aVF (Fig. 1.9). An anterior infarction produces changes mainly in leads V_1 to V_4 (Fig. 1.10).

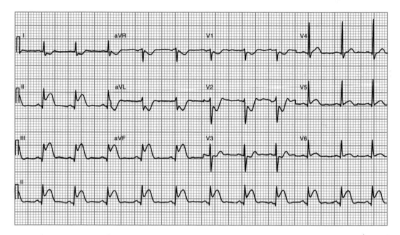

Fig. 1.9 An inferior myocardial infarction produces changes in the inferior leads

Key points: ● leads II, III and aVF look at the inferior surface of the heart

● ST segment elevation is present in these leads (acute inferior myocardial infarction)

● there are also reciprocal changes in leads V_1–V_3, I and aVL

Why are there 12 ECG leads?

Twelve leads simply provide a number of different views of the heart that are manageable (too many leads would take too long to interpret) yet provide a comprehensive picture of the heart's electrical activity (too few leads might 'overlook' important regions). For research purposes, where a more detailed picture of the heart is needed, over 100 leads are often used.

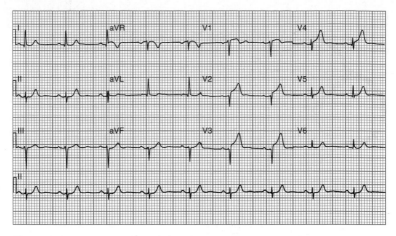

Fig. 1.10 An anterior myocardial infarction produces changes in the anterior leads

Key points: ● leads V_1–V_4 look at the anterior surface of the heart

              ● ST segment elevation is present in these leads, with Q waves in V_1–V_3 (anterior myocardial infarction after 24 h)

WHERE DO THE WAVES COME FROM?

In the normal heart, each beat begins with the discharge ('depolarization') of the sinoatrial (SA) node, high up in the right atrium. This is a spontaneous event, occurring 60–100 times every minute.

Depolarization of the SA node does not cause any noticeable wave on the ECG. The first detectable wave appears when the impulse spreads from the SA node to depolarize the atria (Fig. 1.11). This produces the P **wave**.

The atria contain relatively little muscle, and so the voltage generated by atrial depolarization is relatively small. From the viewpoint of most leads, the electricity appears to flow *towards* them and so the P wave will be a positive (upward) deflection. The exception is lead aVR, where the electricity appears to flow *away*, and so the P wave is negative in that lead (see Fig. 1.8).

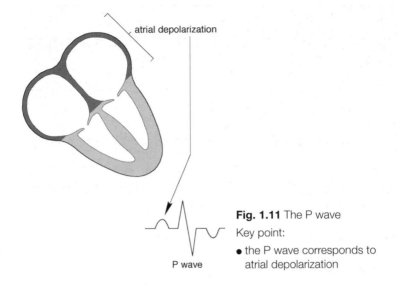

Fig. 1.11 The P wave
Key point:
- the P wave corresponds to atrial depolarization

After flowing through the atria, the electrical impulse reaches the atrioventricular (AV) node, located low in the right atrium. The AV node is normally the only route by which an electrical impulse can reach the ventricles, the rest of the atrial myocardium being separated from the ventricles by a non-conducting ring of fibrous tissue.

Activation of the AV node does not produce an obvious wave on the ECG, but it does contribute to the time interval between the P wave and the subsequent Q or R wave. It does this by delaying conduction, and in doing so acts as a safety mechanism, preventing rapid atrial impulses (for instance during atrial flutter or fibrillation) from spreading to the ventricles at the same rate.

The time taken for the depolarization wave to pass from its origin in the SA node, across the atria, and through the AV node into ventricular muscle is called the **PR interval**. This is measured from the beginning of the P wave to the beginning of the R wave, and is normally between 0.12 and 0.20 s, or 3–5 small squares (Fig. 1.12).

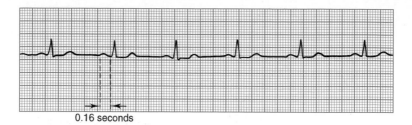

0.16 seconds

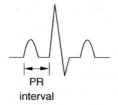

PR interval

Fig. 1.12 The PR interval

Key point:

● the PR interval is normally 0.12–0.20 s long

Once the impulse has traversed the AV node, it enters the bundle of His, a specialized conducting pathway that passes into the interventricular septum and divides into the left and right bundle branches (Fig. 1.13).

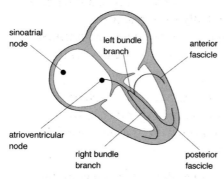

sinoatrial node

left bundle branch

anterior fascicle

atrioventricular node

right bundle branch

posterior fascicle

Fig. 1.13 The right and left bundle branches

Key point:

● the bundle of His divides into right and left bundle branches in the interventricular septum

Current normally flows between the bundle branches in the interventricular septum, from left to right, and this is responsible for the first deflection of the **QRS complex**. Whether this is a downward deflection or an upward deflection depends upon which side of the septum a lead is 'looking' from (Fig. 1.14).

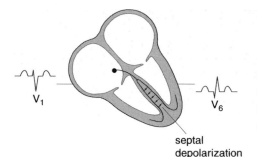

Fig. 1.14 Septal depolarization

Key point:

- the septum normally depolarizes from left to right

septal depolarization

By convention, if the first deflection of the QRS complex is downward, it is called a **Q wave**. The first upward deflection is called an **R wave**, whether or not it follows a Q wave. A downward deflection after an R wave is called an **S wave**. Hence, a variety of complexes is possible (Fig. 1.15).

The right bundle branch conducts the wave of depolarization to the right ventricle, whereas the left bundle branch divides into anterior and posterior fascicles that conduct the wave to the left ventricle (Fig. 1.16). The conducting pathways end by dividing into Purkinje fibres that distribute the wave of depolarization rapidly throughout both ventricles. The depolarization of the ventricles, represented by the QRS complex, is normally complete within 0.12 s (Fig. 1.17).

QRS complexes are 'positive' or 'negative', depending on whether the R wave or the S wave is bigger (Fig. 1.18). This, in turn, will depend upon the view each lead has of the heart.

The left ventricle contains considerably more myocardium than the right, and so the voltage generated by its depolarization will tend to dominate the shape of the QRS complex.

Leads that look at the heart from the right will see a relatively small amount of voltage moving towards them as the right ventricle depolarizes, and a larger amount moving

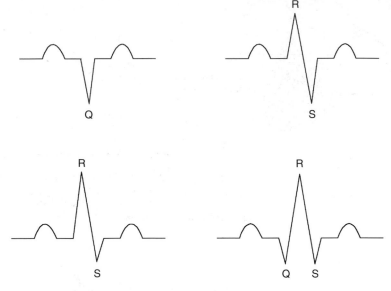

Fig. 1.15 The different varieties of QRS complex

Key points: ● the first downward deflection is a Q wave
● the first upward deflection is an R wave
● a downward deflection after an R wave is an S wave

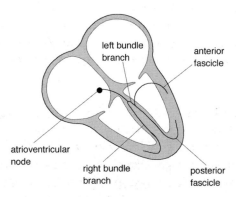

Fig. 1.16 Divisions of the left bundle branch

Key point: ● the left bundle branch divides into anterior and posterior fascicles

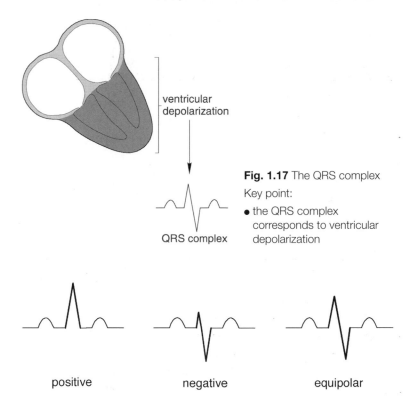

Fig. 1.17 The QRS complex
Key point:
- the QRS complex corresponds to ventricular depolarization

positive   negative   equipolar

Fig. 1.18 Polarity of the QRS complexes
Key points: • a dominant R wave means a positive QRS complex
              • a dominant S wave means a negative QRS complex
              • equal R and S waves mean an equipolar QRS complex

away with depolarization of the left ventricle. The QRS complex will therefore be dominated by an S wave, and be negative. Conversely, leads looking at the heart from the left will see a relatively large voltage moving towards them, and a smaller voltage moving away, giving rise to a large R wave and only a small S wave (Fig. 1.19). Therefore, there is a gradual transition across the chest leads, from a predominantly negative QRS complex to a predominantly positive one (Fig. 1.20).

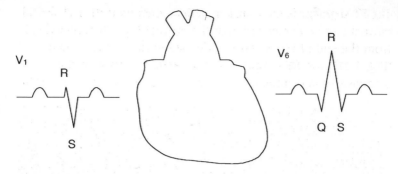

Fig. 1.19 QRS-complex shape varies according to the lead's viewpoint

Key points: • right-sided leads have negative QRS complexes
  • left-sided leads have positive QRS complexes

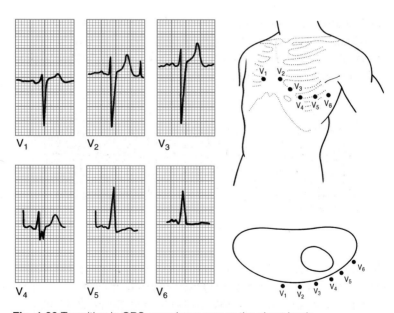

Fig. 1.20 Transition in QRS complexes across the chest leads

Key points: • QRS complexes are normally negative in leads V_1 and V_2

  • QRS complexes are normally positive in leads V_5 and V_6

The **ST segment** is the transient period when no further electrical current can be passed through the myocardium. It is measured from the end of the S wave to the beginning of the T wave (Fig. 1.21). The ST segment is of particular interest in the diagnosis of myocardial infarction and ischaemia (see Chapter 9).

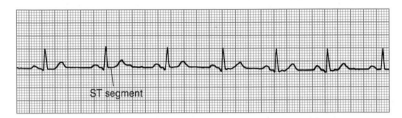

Fig. 1.21 The ST segment

The **T wave** represents repolarization ('recharging') of the ventricular myocardium to its resting electrical state. The **QT interval** measures the total time for activation of the ventricles and recovery to the normal resting state (Fig. 1.22).

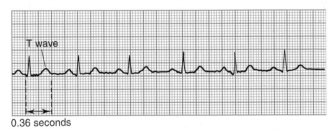

0.36 seconds

Fig. 1.22 The T wave and QT interval

The origin of the **U wave** is uncertain, but it may represent repolarization of the interventricular septum or slow repolarization of the ventricles. U waves can be difficult to identify but, when present, they are most clearly seen in the anterior chest leads V_2–V_4 (Fig. 1.23).

You need to be familiar with the most important electrical events that make up the cardiac cycle. These are summarized at the end of the chapter.

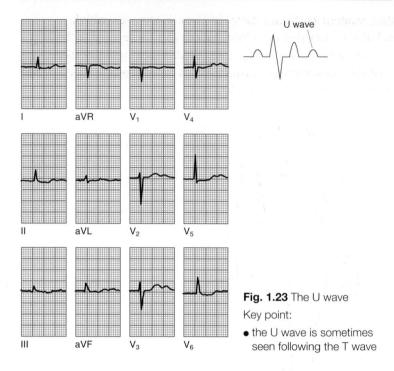

Fig. 1.23 The U wave

Key point:

● the U wave is sometimes seen following the T wave

HOW DO I RECORD AN ECG?

Always ensure you know how to operate the ECG machine before attempting to record an ECG. An incorrect recording can lead to incorrect diagnoses, wasted investigations and potentially disastrous unnecessary treatment.

To record a clear, noise-free ECG, begin by asking the patient to lie down and relax to reduce electrical interference from skeletal muscle. Before attaching the electrodes, prepare the skin underneath with a spirit wipe and remove excess hair to ensure good electrical contact.

Attach the limb and chest electrodes in their correct positions. The limb electrodes are usually labelled and/or colour-coded according to which arm or leg they need to be attached.

Most modern machines have six chest electrodes, which will also be labelled or colour-coded, and these need to be positioned as shown in Fig. 1.24. Older machines may have only one chest electrode, which needs to be repositioned to record each of the six chest leads.

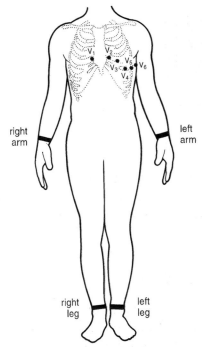

ECG electrodes attached to each limb and to chest

Fig. 1.24 Electrode positions on the limbs and chest

Key point:

● always ensure the electrodes are correctly positioned

When recording the ECG, always check that the machine is properly calibrated so that:

● the paper speed is correct (25 mm/s is standard)
● the calibration mark has been made, such that 10 mm = 1 mV, so that wave height can readily be converted into a more meaningful voltage.

The recognition of artefacts on the ECG is discussed in Chapter 13.

Summary

The waves and intervals of the ECG correspond to the following events:

ECG event	Cardiac event
P wave	Atrial depolarization
PR interval	Start of atrial depolarization to start of ventricular depolarization
QRS complex	Ventricular depolarization
ST segment	Pause in ventricular electrical activity before repolarization
T wave	Ventricular repolarization
QT interval	Total time taken by ventricular depolarization and repolarization
U wave	Uncertain – possibly: • interventricular septal repolarization • slow ventricular repolarization

Note. Depolarizations of the SA and AV nodes are important events but do not *in themselves* produce a detectable wave on the standard ECG.

2

HEART RATE

$\mathbf{M}$easurement of the heart rate and the identification of the cardiac rhythm go hand in hand, as many abnormalities of heart rate result from arrhythmias. How to identify the cardiac rhythm is discussed in detail in the following chapter. To begin with, however, we will simply describe ways to measure the heart rate and the abnormalities that can affect it.

When we talk of measuring the heart rate, we usually mean the *ventricular* rate, which corresponds to the patient's pulse. Depolarization of the ventricles produces the QRS complex on the ECG, and so it is the rate of QRS complexes that we want to measure to determine the heart rate.

Measurement of the heart rate is simple and can be done in several ways. Before you try to measure anything, however, check that the ECG has been recorded at the standard UK and USA paper speed of 25 mm/s. If so, then all you have to remember is that a 1-min ECG tracing covers **300 large squares**. If the patient's rhythm is regular, all you have to do is count the number of large squares between two QRS complexes, and divide it into 300.

For example, in Fig. 2.1 there are 5 large squares between each QRS complex. Therefore:

$$\text{Heart rate} = \frac{300}{5} = 60/\text{min}$$

This method does not work so well when the rhythm is irregular, as the number of large squares between each QRS

5 large squares

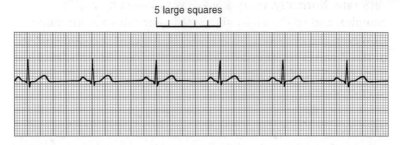

Fig. 2.1 Calculating heart rate when the rhythm is regular

Key points: ● 1 QRS complex every 5 large squares

  ● 300 large squares correspond to 1 min

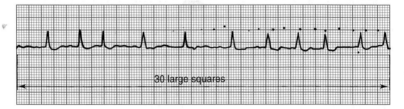

30 large squares

Fig. 2.2 Calculating heart rate when the rhythm is irregular

Key points: ● 30 large squares contain 11 QRS complexes

  ● 30 large squares correspond to 6 s

complex varies from beat to beat. Instead, count the number of QRS complexes in 30 large squares (Fig. 2.2). This is the number of QRS complexes in 6 s. To work out the rate/min, simply multiply by 10:

Number of QRS complexes in 30 squares = 11
Therefore, number of QRS complexes in 6 s = 11
Therefore, number of QRS complexes/min = 11 × 10 = 110

An ECG ruler can be helpful, but follow the instructions on it carefully. Some ECG machines will calculate heart rate and print it on the ECG, but always check machine-derived values, as machines do occasionally make errors!

Whichever method you use, remember it can also be used to measure the atrial or P wave rate as well as the ventricular or

QRS rate. Normally, every P wave is followed by a QRS complex and so the atrial and ventricular rates are the same. However, the rates can be different if, for example, some or all of the P waves are prevented from activating the ventricles (Fig. 2.3). Situations where this may happen are described in later chapters.

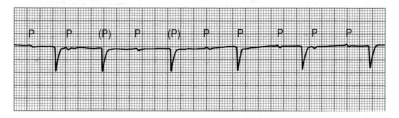

Fig. 2.3 The P wave rate can differ from the QRS complex rate
Key points: ● P wave (atrial) rate is 105/min
            ● QRS complex (ventricular) rate is 60/min

Once you have measured the heart rate, you need to decide whether it is normal or abnormal. As a general rule, a regular heart rhythm with a rate between 60 and 100 beats/min is normal. If the rate is below 60 beats/min, the patient is said to be **bradycardic**. With a heart rate above 100 beats/min, the patient is **tachycardic**. Therefore, the two questions you need to ask about heart rate are:

● Is the heart rate below 60 beats/min?
● Is the heart rate above 100 beats/min?

If the answer to either question is 'yes', turn to the appropriate half of this chapter to find out what to do next. If not, turn to Chapter 3 to identify the cardiac rhythm.

IS THE HEART RATE BELOW 60 BEATS PER MINUTE?

Bradycardia is arbitrarily defined as a heart rate below 60 beats/min. Identification of the cardiac rhythm and any conduction disturbances is essential, and help with this can be found in Chapter 3.

Problems to consider in the bradycardic patient are:

- sinus bradycardia
- sick sinus syndrome
- second-degree and third-degree atrioventricular (AV) block
- 'escape' rhythms
  - AV junctional escape rhythm
  - ventricular escape rhythms
  - asystole.

Sinus bradycardia (p. 32) can be normal, for example in athletes during sleep, but in others may indicate an underlying problem. The differential diagnosis and treatment are discussed in Chapter 3.

Sick sinus syndrome (p. 35) is the coexistence of sinus bradycardia with episodes of sinus arrest and sinoatrial block. Patients may also have episodes of paroxysmal tachycardia, giving rise to the tachy-brady syndrome.

In **second-degree AV block** (p. 117) some atrial impulses fail to be conducted to the ventricles, and this can lead to bradycardia. In **third-degree AV block**, no atrial impulses can reach the ventricles; in response, the ventricles usually develop an 'escape' rhythm (see below). It is important to remember that AV block can coexist with *any* atrial rhythm.

Escape rhythms (p. 58) are a form of 'safety net' to maintain a heart beat if the normal mechanism of impulse generation fails or is blocked. They may also appear during episodes of severe sinus bradycardia. The distinction between AV junctional and ventricular escape rhythms is discussed in Chapter 3.

Asystole (p. 250) implies the absence of ventricular activity, and so the heart rate is zero. Asystole is a medical emergency and requires immediate diagnosis and treatment if the patient is to survive. A management algorithm can be found in Fig. 17.5.

Table 2.1 Negatively chronotropic drugs

Beta blockers (do not forget eye drops)
Some calcium antagonists, e.g. verapamil, diltiazem
Digoxin
Adenosine

Don't forget that arrhythmias that are usually associated with normal or fast heart rates may be slowed by certain drugs, resulting in bradycardia. For example, patients with atrial fibrillation (which, untreated, causes a *tachycardia*) can develop a *bradycardia* when commenced on anti-arrhythmic drugs. Drugs that commonly slow the heart rate (**negatively chronotropic**) are listed in Table 2.1. A thorough review of all the patient's current and recent medications is therefore essential.

 DRUG POINT

A complete drug history is essential in any patient with an abnormal ECG.

The first step in managing a bradycardia is to assess the urgency of the situation. Ask the patient about symptoms (dizziness, syncope, falls, fatigue, breathlessness, chest pain and palpitations) and perform a thorough examination, looking particularly for evidence of haemodynamic disturbance (hypotension, cardiac failure and poor peripheral perfusion).

Use the history, examination and further investigations (e.g. plasma electrolytes, thyroid function tests) to identify any underlying cause, and correct it where possible:

- Discontinue or reduce the dose of responsible drugs.
- Identify abnormal cardiac rhythms.
- Identify and treat hypothyroidism.

When bradycardia is severe and symptomatic, more urgent treatment is required:

- atropine 300–600 mcg given slowly intravenously (do not exceed 3 mg in 24 h).

However, if a pacemaker is likely to be needed (see Chapter 14), atropine should only be used as a short-term measure while arranging for temporary pacing.

Chronic bradycardia may be an indication for a permanent pacemaker, particularly when it is causing symptoms or haemodynamic disturbance. Referral to a cardiologist is recommended.

SEEK HELP

Bradycardias may require pacing, especially if symptomatic. Seek the advice of a cardiologist, without delay.

IS THE HEART RATE ABOVE 100 BEATS PER MINUTE?

Tachycardia is arbitrarily defined as a heart rate above 100 beats/min. When a patient presents with a tachycardia, you must begin by identifying the cardiac rhythm. Consult Chapter 3 for specific descriptions of how to recognize and manage each rhythm.

You can begin the process of identification by checking whether the QRS complexes are:

- narrow (<3 small squares)
- broad (>3 small squares).

Narrow-complex tachycardias always arise from above the ventricles; that is, they are supraventricular in origin. The possibilities are:

- sinus tachycardia
- atrial tachycardia
- atrial flutter
- atrial fibrillation
- AV re-entry tachycardias.

All of these are discussed in detail in Chapter 3.

Broad QRS complexes can occur if normal electrical impulses are conducted abnormally or 'aberrantly' to the ventricles. This delays ventricular activation, widening the QRS complex. Any of the supraventricular tachycardias (SVTs) listed above can also present as a **broad-complex tachycardia** if aberrant conduction is present.

Broad-complex tachycardia should also make you think of ventricular arrhythmias:

- ventricular tachycardia
- accelerated idioventricular rhythm
- torsades de pointes.

Each of these is discussed in Chapter 3, and advice on how to distinguish between ventricular tachycardia and SVT can be found on p. 73.

Ventricular fibrillation (VF) is hard to categorize. The chaotic nature of the underlying ventricular activity can give rise to a variety of ECG appearances, but all have the characteristics of being unpredictable and chaotic. VF is a medical emergency and so it is important that you can recognize it immediately; you should study Chapter 17 if you are not confident in doing so.

The management of tachycardia depends upon the underlying rhythm, and the treatment of the different arrhythmias is detailed in Chapter 3. The first step, as with managing a bradycardia, is to assess the urgency of the situation.

Clues to the nature of the arrhythmia may be found in the patient's history. Ask the patient about how any palpitations start and stop (sudden or gradual), whether there are any situations in which they are more likely to happen (e.g. during exercise, lying quietly in bed), how long they last and whether there are any associated symptoms (dizziness, syncope, falls, fatigue, breathlessness and chest pain). Also ask the patient to 'tap out' how the palpitations feel – this will give you clues as to the rate (fast or slow) and rhythm (regular or irregular).

You must also enquire about symptoms of related disorders (e.g. hyperthyroidism) and obtain a list of current medications. Check for any drugs (e.g. salbutamol) that can increase the heart rate (**positively chronotropic**). Do not forget to ask about caffeine intake (coffee, tea and cola drinks).

A thorough examination is always important, looking for evidence of haemodynamic disturbance (hypotension, cardiac failure and poor peripheral perfusion) and coexistent disorders (e.g. a thyroid goitre).

Use the history, examination and further investigations (e.g. plasma electrolytes, thyroid function tests) to reach a diagnosis. Ambulatory ECG recording may be helpful if circumstances permit it (see Chapter 15).

In an emergency, every effort must be made to diagnose and correct the rhythm as quickly as possible. If the diagnosis is unclear and the patient needs immediate treatment, most tachycardias will respond to direct current cardioversion. Do not hesitate to seek the urgent advice of a cardiologist if circumstances permit.

 ACT QUICKLY

Tachycardia causing haemodynamic disturbance requires urgent diagnosis and treatment.

Summary

To assess the heart rate, ask the following questions.

1. Is the heart rate below 60 beats/min?

If 'yes', consider:
- sinus bradycardia
- sick sinus syndrome
- second-degree and third-degree AV block
- escape rhythms
  - AV junctional escape rhythm
  - ventricular escape rhythms
  - asystole
  - drug-induced condition.

2. Is the heart rate above 100 beats/min?

If 'yes', consider:
- narrow-complex tachycardia
  - sinus tachycardia
  - atrial tachycardia
  - atrial flutter
  - atrial fibrillation
  - AV re-entry tachycardias
- broad-complex tachycardia
  - narrow-complex tachycardia with aberrant conduction
  - ventricular tachycardia
  - accelerated idioventricular rhythm
  - torsades de pointes.

3

RHYTHM

To identify the cardiac rhythm with confidence you need to examine a rhythm strip – a prolonged recording of the ECG from just one lead, usually lead II (Fig. 3.1). Most modern ECG machines automatically include a rhythm strip at the bottom of a 12-lead ECG. If your machine does not, make sure you have recorded one yourself. The diagnosis of rhythm abnormalities may only become apparent when you examine 12 or more consecutive complexes.

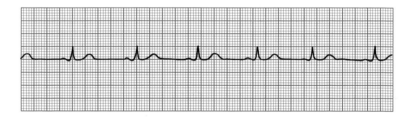

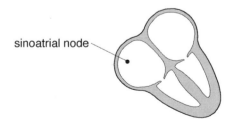

sinoatrial node

Fig. 3.1 The rhythm strip
Key points:
- rhythm strips are prolonged recordings from a single lead, often lead II
- this rhythm strip shows sinus rhythm

Even with a rhythm strip, however, the diagnosis of abnormal cardiac rhythms is not always easy, and some of the more complex arrhythmias can tax the skills of even the most experienced cardiologist. It is appropriate, therefore, to begin this chapter with the following warning.

 SEEK HELP

If in doubt about a patient's cardiac rhythm, do not hesitate to seek the advice of a cardiologist.

This advice is particularly important if the patient is haemodynamically compromised by the arrhythmia, or if you are contemplating treatment of any kind.

There are many ways in which one can approach the identification of arrhythmias, and this is reflected in the numerous ways in which they can be categorized:

● regular vs irregular
● bradycardias vs tachycardias
● narrow complex vs broad complex
● supraventricular vs ventricular.

The common cardiac rhythms are listed in Table 3.1. The first half of this chapter contains a brief description of each rhythm in turn, together with example ECGs. In the second half, 'Identifying the cardiac rhythm', we guide you towards the correct diagnosis of the cardiac rhythm.

SINUS RHYTHM

Sinus rhythm is the normal cardiac rhythm, in which the sinoatrial (SA) node acts as the natural pacemaker, discharging 60–100 times/min (Fig. 3.2).

The characteristic features of sinus rhythm are:

● the heart rate is 60–100 beats/min
● the P wave is upright in lead II and inverted in lead aVR
● every P wave is followed by a QRS complex.

Table 3.1 Cardiac rhythms

- SA nodal rhythms
  - sinus rhythm
  - sinus bradycardia
  - sinus tachycardia
  - sinus arrhythmia
  - sick sinus syndrome
- Atrial rhythms
  - atrial tachycardia
  - atrial flutter
  - atrial fibrillation
  - AV junctional rhythms
  - AV re-entry tachycardias
- Ventricular rhythms
  - ventricular tachycardia
  - accelerated idioventricular rhythm
  - torsades de pointes
  - ventricular fibrillation
- Conduction disturbances
- Escape rhythms
- Ectopic beats

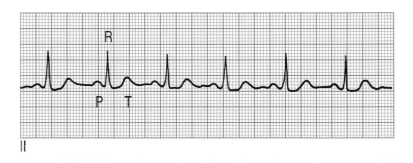

II

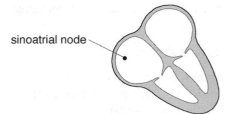

sinoatrial node

Fig. 3.2 Sinus rhythm

Key points:

- heart rate is 80 beats/min
- P waves are upright (lead II)
- QRS complex after every P wave

If the patient is in sinus rhythm, move on to determine the cardiac axis (Chapter 4). If not, continue reading this chapter to diagnose the rhythm.

SINUS BRADYCARDIA

Sinus bradycardia is sinus rhythm with a heart rate of less than 60 beats/min (Fig. 3.3).

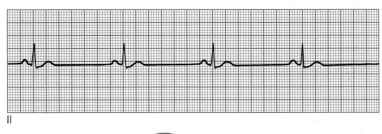

II

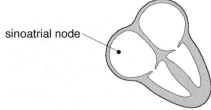

sinoatrial node

Fig. 3.3 Sinus bradycardia
Key points:
- heart rate is 43 beats/min
- P waves are upright (lead II)
- QRS complex after every P wave

The characteristic features of sinus bradycardia are:

- the heart rate is *less than* 60 beats/min
- the P wave is upright in lead II and inverted in lead aVR
- every P wave is followed by a QRS complex.

It is unusual for sinus bradycardia to be slower than 40 beats/min – any slower and you should consider an alternative cause, such as heart block (p. 116). Sinus bradycardia can be a normal finding, for example in athletes or during sleep. However, always consider the following possible causes:

- drugs (e.g. digoxin, beta blockers – including eye drops)
- ischaemic heart disease and myocardial infarction
- hypothyroidism

- hypothermia
- electrolyte abnormalities
- obstructive jaundice
- uraemia
- raised intracranial pressure
- sick sinus syndrome.

If the sinus bradycardia is severe, or if sinus arrest or SA block is prolonged, escape beats and escape rhythms may occur.

The management of bradycardia (of any cause) is discussed in detail in Chapter 2.

SINUS TACHYCARDIA

Sinus tachycardia is sinus rhythm with a heart rate of greater than 100 beats/min (Fig. 3.4).

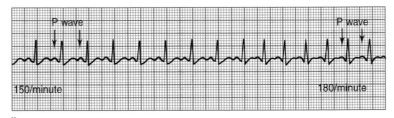

II

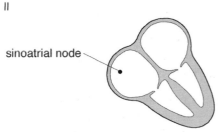

sinoatrial node

Fig. 3.4 Sinus tachycardia
Key points:

- heart rate is 150–180 beats/min
- P waves are upright (lead II)
- QRS complex after every P wave

The characteristic features of sinus tachycardia are:

- the heart rate is *greater than* 100 beats/min
- the P wave is upright in lead II and inverted in lead aVR
- every P wave is followed by a QRS complex.

It is rare for sinus tachycardia to exceed 180 beats/min, except in fit athletes. At this heart rate, it may be difficult to differentiate the P waves from the T waves, so the rhythm can be mistaken for an atrioventricular (AV) nodal re-entry tachycardia.

Physiological causes of a sinus tachycardia include anything that stimulates the sympathetic nervous system – anxiety, pain, fear, fever or exercise. Always consider the following causes too:

- drugs, e.g. adrenaline, atropine, salbutamol (do not forget inhalers and nebulizers), caffeine and alcohol
- ischaemic heart disease and acute myocardial infarction
- heart failure
- pulmonary embolism
- fluid loss
- anaemia
- hyperthyroidism.

The management of sinus tachycardia is that of the cause. When a patient has an **appropriate** tachycardia (compensating for low blood pressure, such as in fluid loss or anaemia), slowing it with beta blockers can lead to disastrous decompensation. It is the underlying problem that needs addressing. However, if the sinus tachycardia is **inappropriate**, as in anxiety or hyperthyroidism, treatment with beta blockers may be helpful.

 WARNING

In sinus tachycardia, never use a beta blocker to slow the heart rate until you have established the cause.

Persistent 'sinus tachycardia' should lead to suspicion that the diagnosis may be incorrect – both atrial flutter and atrial tachycardia can, on casual inspection, be mistaken for sinus tachycardia. In very rare cases it is possible for sinus tachycardia to result from a re-entry circuit within the SA node. In such cases the tachycardia can usually be terminated with vagal manoeuvres (such as the Valsalva manoeuvre – see below).

SINUS ARRHYTHMIA

Sinus arrhythmia is the variation in heart rate that is seen during inspiration and expiration (Fig. 3.5).

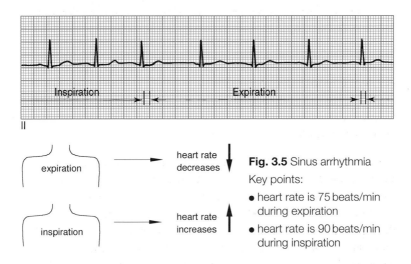

Fig. 3.5 Sinus arrhythmia
Key points:
- heart rate is 75 beats/min during expiration
- heart rate is 90 beats/min during inspiration

The characteristic features of sinus arrhythmia are:

- every P wave is followed by a QRS complex
- the heart rate varies with respiration.

The heart rate normally increases during inspiration, as a reflex response to the increased volume of blood returning to the heart. Sinus arrhythmia is uncommon after the age of 40 years. The condition is harmless and no tests or treatment are necessary.

SICK SINUS SYNDROME

As the name suggests, sick sinus syndrome is a collection of impulse generation and conduction problems related to dysfunction of the sinus node. Any, or all, of the following problems may be seen in a patient with the syndrome:

- sinus bradycardia
- sinus arrest
- SA block.

Sinus bradycardia has already been described (p. 32). The sinus node is normally a very reliable pacemaker. However, in **sinus arrest**, it sometimes fails to discharge on time – looking at a rhythm strip, a P wave will suddenly fail to appear in the expected place, and there is a gap, of variable length, until the sinus node fires and a P wave appears (Fig. 3.6).

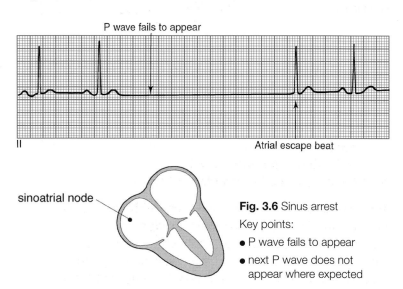

P wave fails to appear

II   Atrial escape beat

sinoatrial node

Fig. 3.6 Sinus arrest
Key points:
- P wave fails to appear
- next P wave does not appear where expected

In **sinoatrial block**, the sinus node depolarizes as normal, but the impulse fails to reach the atria. A P wave fails to appear in the expected place, but the next one usually appears exactly where it is expected (Fig. 3.7).

If the sinus bradycardia is severe, or if sinus arrest or SA block is prolonged, escape beats and escape

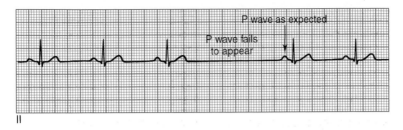

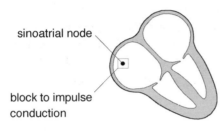

sinoatrial node

block to impulse
conduction

Fig. 3.7 Sinoatrial block
Key points:
- P wave fails to appear
- next P wave appears where expected

rhythms may occur. Sick sinus syndrome may also coexist with:

- certain paroxysmal tachycardias
  - atrial tachycardia (p. 38)
  - atrial flutter (p. 40)
  - atrial fibrillation (AF) (p. 43)
- AV nodal conduction disorders (p. 116).

The association of sick sinus syndrome with paroxysmal tachycardias is called **tachycardia–bradycardia (or 'tachy-brady') syndrome**. The tachycardias often emerge as an escape rhythm in response to an episode of bradycardia. Evidence for abnormal AV nodal conduction often becomes apparent when a patient with tachy-brady syndrome develops AF with a slow ventricular response – the AV node fails to conduct the atrial impulses at the usual high rate.

Sick sinus syndrome, and the associated tachy-brady syndrome, may cause symptoms of dizziness, fainting and palpitations. The commonest cause of sick sinus syndrome is degeneration and fibrosis of the sinus node and conducting system. Other causes to consider are:

- ischaemic heart disease
- drugs (e.g. digoxin, quinidine, beta blockers)
- cardiomyopathy
- amyloidosis
- myocarditis.

The diagnosis usually requires a 24-h ambulatory ECG recording, also known as **Holter monitoring** (see Chapter 15).

Asymptomatic patients do not require treatment. Symptomatic patients need consideration for a permanent pacemaker (Chapter 14). This is particularly important if they also have paroxysmal tachycardias that require anti-arrhythmic drugs (which can worsen the episodes of bradycardia). Paroxysmal tachycardias that arise as escape rhythms in response to episodes of bradycardia may also improve as a consequence of pacing. Referral to a cardiologist is therefore recommended.

ATRIAL TACHYCARDIA

Atrial tachycardia differs from sinus tachycardia in that the impulses are generated by an ectopic focus somewhere within the atrial myocardium rather than the sinus node (Fig. 3.8).

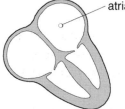
— atrial ectopic focus

Fig. 3.8 Abnormal atrial focus
Key point:

- the abnormal focus means the spread of depolarization through the atria follows an abnormal route

This results in a rhythm strip with the following characteristic features (Fig. 3.9):

- heart rate greater than 100 beats/min
- abnormally shaped P waves.

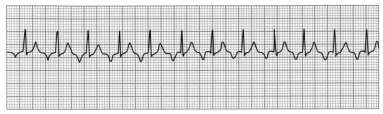

II

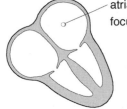

atrial ectopic
focus

Fig. 3.9 Atrial tachycardia
Key points:
● heart rate is 125 beats/min
● abnormally shaped P waves

The atrial (P wave) rate is usually 120–250/min; above atrial rates of 200/min, the AV node struggles to keep up with impulse conduction and AV block may occur. The combination of atrial tachycardia with AV block is particularly common in digoxin toxicity. If the patient is not taking digoxin, consider:

● ischaemic heart disease
● rheumatic heart disease
● cardiomyopathy
● sick sinus syndrome (p. 35)
● chronic obstructive pulmonary disease.

For details on how to manage digoxin toxicity, see the section on digoxin in Chapter 9 (p. 173). If digoxin is not the cause, it can be used to control the ventricular response, as can a beta blocker or verapamil.

 WARNING

Never give verapamil to a patient who is taking a beta blocker (or vice versa). A severe bradycardia can result.

ATRIAL FLUTTER

Atrial flutter usually results from a re-entry circuit within the right atrium. It takes around 0.2 s for the impulse to complete a circuit of the right atrium, giving rise to a wave of depolarization across both atria and a flutter wave on the ECG. There are thus around 5 flutter waves every second, and around 300 every minute (Fig. 3.10).

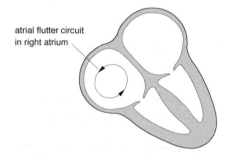

atrial flutter circuit
in right atrium

Fig. 3.10 Atrial flutter circuit
Key point:
- a circuit of activity circles the right atrium

In atrial flutter the atrial rate is usually 250–350/min and often almost exactly 300/min. The AV node cannot keep up with such a high atrial rate and AV block occurs. This is most commonly 2:1 block, where only alternate atrial impulses get through the AV node to initiate a QRS complex, although 3:1, 4:1 or variable degrees of block are also seen (Fig. 3.11).

Thus, the ventricular rate is less than the atrial rate, and is often 150, 100 or 75/min. You should always suspect atrial flutter with 2:1 block when a patient has a regular tachycardia with a ventricular rate of around 150/min.

The rapid atrial rate gives a characteristic 'sawtooth' appearance to the baseline of the ECG, made up of flutter or 'F' waves. This can be made more apparent by carotid sinus massage or by giving adenosine. This will not terminate the atrial flutter, but will increase the degree of AV block, making the baseline easier to see by reducing the number of QRS complexes (Fig. 3.12).

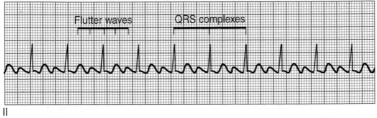

Flutter waves   QRS complexes

II

atrial flutter circuit
in right atrium

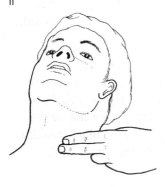

AV node

intermittent block
of AV node

Fig. 3.11 Atrial flutter with 3:1
AV block

Key points:

- flutter waves at a rate of 300/min
- QRS complexes at a rate of 100/min
- therefore, 3:1 AV block is present

Carotid sinus
massage

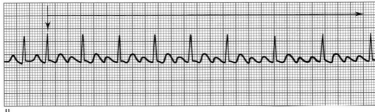

II

Fig. 3.12 The effect of carotid sinus
massage

Key points:

- carotid sinus massage increases
  the degree of AV block
- the QRS rate falls from 100/min to
  75/min
- the flutter waves are more easily seen
  when there are fewer QRS complexes

Thus, the characteristic features of atrial flutter are:

- atrial rate around 300/min
- 'sawtooth' baseline
- AV block (usually 2:1, 3:1 or 4:1).

The causes of atrial flutter are the same as those of AF (see Table 3.2). Although beta blockers, verapamil or digoxin can be used simply to control the ventricular response, it is preferable to aim to restore sinus rhythm. Drugs that can restore (and maintain) sinus rhythm include:

- sotalol
- flecainide
- propafenone.

Table 3.2 Causes of atrial fibrillation

- Hypertension
- Ischaemic heart disease
- Hyperthyroidism
- Sick sinus syndrome
- Alcohol
- Rheumatic mitral valve disease
- Cardiomyopathy
- Atrial septal defect
- Pericarditis
- Myocarditis
- Pulmonary embolism
- Pneumonia
- Cardiac surgery
- Idiopathic ('lone') atrial fibrillation

Atrial flutter can also be converted to sinus rhythm with direct current (DC) cardioversion (p. 14) and overdrive atrial pacing (Chapter 14). Atrial flutter ablation can be used to prevent recurrence of the arrhythmia. This is an electrophysiological technique in which the re-entry circuit is identified in the right atrium and a section of it is permanently ablated using diathermy to 'break' the circuit underlying the re-entry loop.

ATRIAL FIBRILLATION

Atrial fibrillation is much commoner than atrial flutter, affecting 5–10 per cent of elderly people. It can be classified as permanent, persistent or paroxysmal.

● **Paroxysmal AF** – spontaneously terminating episodes of AF on a background of sinus rhythm.
● **Persistent AF** – continuous AF with no intervening sinus rhythm.
● **Permanent AF** – continuous AF where there is no expectation of restoring sinus rhythm (e.g. by DC cardioversion).

The basis of AF is rapid, chaotic depolarization occurring throughout the atria as a consequence of multiple 'wavelets' of activation. No P waves are seen and the ECG baseline consists of low-amplitude oscillations (fibrillation or 'f' waves). Although around 350–600 impulses reach the AV node every minute, only 120–180 of these will reach the ventricles to produce QRS complexes. Transmission of the atrial impulses through the AV node is erratic, making the ventricular (QRS complex) rhythm 'irregularly irregular' (Fig. 3.13).

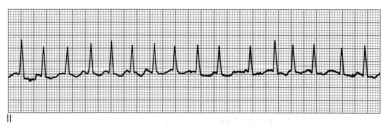

II

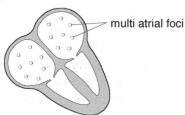

multi atrial foci

Fig. 3.13 Atrial fibrillation
Key points:
● irregularly irregular rhythm
● no P waves visible
● QRS rate is 170/min

Thus, the characteristic features of AF are:

● absence of P waves
● irregularly irregular ventricular rhythm.

The erratic atrial depolarization leads to a failure of effective atrial contraction. Loss of the 'atrial kick' reduces ventricular filling and can lead to a fall of 10–15 per cent in cardiac output.

Patients with AF usually present with palpitations and/or symptoms of an underlying cause (Table 3.2). Systemic embolism is a significant risk in AF and may also be a presenting feature. Examination of the patient will reveal an irregularly irregular pulse.

Once AF has been diagnosed, a cause should be sought with a thorough patient history and examination. Thyroid function tests are essential, as AF may be the only sign of a thyroid disorder. Echocardiography may also be helpful. Treatment of an underlying cause can resolve the arrhythmia.

In treating permanent AF, aim to:

● control the ventricular rate
● reduce the risk of thromboembolism
● restore sinus rhythm (if possible).

Rate control is achieved with AV nodal blocking drugs, such as beta blockers, verapamil or digoxin.

! WARNING

Never give verapamil to a patient who is taking a beta blocker (or vice versa). A severe bradycardia can result.

The risk of stroke in AF is reduced by about 60 per cent with anticoagulation treatment using warfarin. However, the indications for anticoagulation in non-rheumatic AF remain controversial. Patients without risk factors for thromboembolic events may require only aspirin. Risk factors include previous thromboembolic episode, age 65 or over, hypertension, diabetes mellitus, heart failure, large left atrium or impaired left ventricular function. The use of warfarin is most controversial in the elderly, who have the highest risk of stroke but also the highest risk of bleeding when taking warfarin. The benefits and risks of anticoagulation for AF must always be weighed up before initiating treatment.

Direct current cardioversion for atrial fibrillation

Although DC cardioversion for AF is often initially successful in restoring sinus rhythm, the arrhythmia frequently recurs. Long-term success is more likely if patients have been in AF for only a short time and if the atria are not significantly enlarged.

Four weeks of full anticoagulation prior to elective DC cardioversion reduces thromboembolic risk. Oral digoxin need not be routinely stopped prior to the procedure, although there is a risk of precipitating a ventricular arrhythmia if digoxin toxicity is present.

Patients must be 'nil by mouth' on the day of the procedure as they will require general anaesthesia. Check their electrolyte levels and INR. The patient should be fully anticoagulated and the plasma potassium level should be >4 mmol/L. If there is a possibility of digoxin toxicity (suggested by symptoms, ECG findings, high dosage or renal impairment), check the patient's digoxin level.

The technique of giving a DC shock is described in Chapter 17. Set the defibrillator to synchronized mode and start at an energy level of 100 J, increasing to 200 J and 360 J as appropriate. In atrial flutter, start at a lower energy level of 50 J. The newer biphasic defibrillators also require lower energy levels.

If cardioversion is successful, continue anticoagulation and review the patient, in clinic, after 4 weeks. If they are still in sinus rhythm, anticoagulation can then be discontinued.

A permanent restoration of sinus rhythm can be difficult to achieve, particularly in patients who have been in AF for a long time. Certain drugs (sotalol, flecainide, propafenone and quinidine) can restore sinus rhythm, as can DC cardioversion (see box above). Maintenance of sinus rhythm can be achieved with any of these drugs, but there is only around a 50:50 chance of sustaining sinus rhythm beyond 1 year. Amiodarone is probably more effective, but can lead to troublesome side-effects.

In paroxysmal AF, the aim should be to reduce embolization risk (as above) and to reduce the likelihood of recurrent paroxysms. Sotalol, flecainide, propafenone and disopyramide may each be useful. Digoxin should be avoided as it does not help in paroxysmal AF, and may even make it worse.

Patients whose AF is resistant to treatment should be referred to a cardiologist.

Resistant atrial fibrillation

The non-pharmacological treatment of resistant AF includes:

- AV nodal ablation (to prevent conduction from the atria to the ventricles) with insertion of a permanent ventricular pacemaker;
- experimental surgical techniques to remodel the atrial myocardium to redirect the flow of atrial impulses.

AV RE-ENTRY TACHYCARDIAS

AV re-entry tachycardias can arise when there is a second connection between the atria and ventricles, in addition to the normal route of conduction via the AV node. The presence of two different routes creates the possibility that impulses can travel down one (anterograde conduction) and then back up the other (retrograde conduction). In doing so, an impulse can enter into a repeated cycle of activity, circling round the two pathways so that it repeatedly re-enters and activates the atria and ventricles in rapid succession (Fig. 3.14).

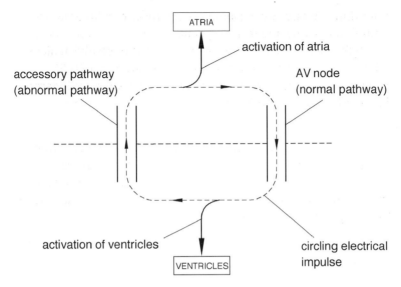

Fig. 3.14 Conduction around an AV re-entry circuit

The extra connection between atria and ventricles can be either an **accessory pathway,** anatomically separate from the AV node, or a **dual AV nodal pathway,** in which both pathways lie within the AV node but are electrically distinct (Fig. 3.15).

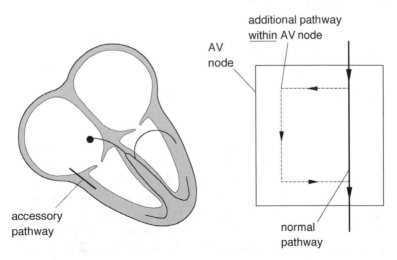

Fig. 3.15 Accessory and dual AV nodal pathways

Accessory pathways are found in the Wolff–Parkinson–White (WPW) syndrome (described in Chapter 6) and patients are susceptible to episodes of **AV re-entry tachycardia,** with anterograde conduction via the AV node and retrograde conduction via the accessory pathway. During the tachycardia the delta wave is lost (Fig. 3.16). A re-entrant tachycardia taking the opposite route (down the accessory pathway and up the AV node) is very rare, but when it does occur, only delta waves are seen (as the whole of the ventricular muscle is activated via the accessory pathway).

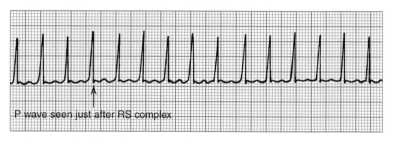

P wave seen just after RS complex

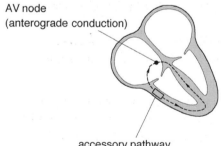

AV node
(anterograde conduction)

accessory pathway
(retrograde conduction)

Fig. 3.16 AV re-entry tachycardia in WPW syndrome
Key points:
● ventricular rate is 188/min
● narrow RS complexes

Patients with a dual AV nodal pathway are at risk of **AV nodal re-entry tachycardia,** in which anterograde conduction usually occurs down the normal AV nodal pathway and returns retrogradely via the abnormal additional pathway (Fig. 3.17).

Both AV re-entry tachycardia and AV nodal re-entry tachycardia have the following characteristics:

● the heart rate is 130–250 beats/min

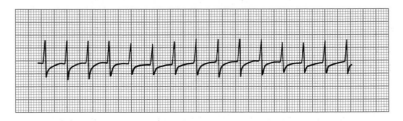

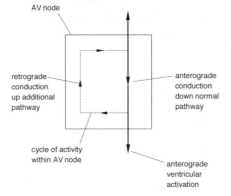

AV node

retrograde conduction up additional pathway

anterograde conduction down normal pathway

cycle of activity within AV node

anterograde ventricular activation

Fig. 3.17 AV nodal re-entry tachycardia

Key points:

- ventricular rate is 180/min
- narrow RS complexes

- there is one P wave per QRS complex (although P waves are not always clearly seen)
- there are regular QRS complexes
- QRS complexes are narrow (in the absence of aberrant conduction).

The QRS complexes will be broad if there is pre-existing or rate-dependent bundle branch block. The rhythm can then be mistaken for ventricular tachycardia (VT) (p. 52). An earlier ECG, if available, may be helpful in determining whether a bundle branch block existed before the tachycardia (Fig. 3.18).

In AV re-entry tachycardia, inverted P waves (p. 102) are often seen halfway between QRS complexes. In AV nodal re-entry tachycardia, the inverted P waves are often harder or even impossible to discern as they follow the QRS complexes closely or are buried within them.

Although the position of the P waves may help distinguish between AV re-entry tachycardia and AV nodal re-entry

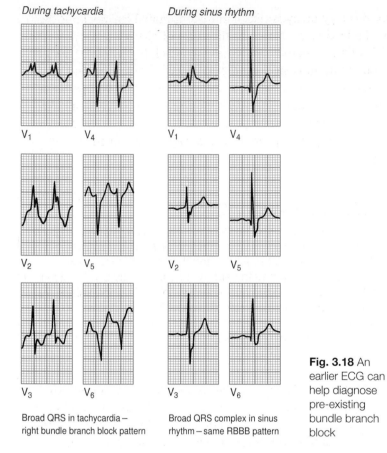

During tachycardia

V_1 V_4

V_2 V_5

V_3 V_6

Broad QRS in tachycardia –
right bundle branch block pattern

During sinus rhythm

V_1 V_4

V_2 V_5

V_3 V_6

Broad QRS complex in sinus
rhythm – same RBBB pattern

Fig. 3.18 An earlier ECG can help diagnose pre-existing bundle branch block

tachycardia, an ECG in sinus rhythm is more helpful as it may reveal a short PR interval or delta wave, suggesting WPW syndrome (p. 111). The definite diagnosis can be difficult, however, and sometimes requires electrophysiological studies.

Symptoms of AV re-entry tachycardias are very variable amongst patients. Palpitations are the commonest complaint, and can vary greatly in duration and severity. They start suddenly and may be accompanied by chest pain, dizziness or syncope.

AV re-entry tachycardias can be terminated by blocking the AV node, thereby breaking the cycle of electrical activity. The **Valsalva manoeuvre** increases vagal inhibition of AV nodal conduction, thus slowing the AV nodal conduction and often terminating the tachycardia. Alternatively, you can perform **carotid sinus massage** (while monitoring the ECG) with the same aim, as long as the patient does not have carotid bruits. The technique of carotid sinus massage is illustrated in Fig. 3.12.

Valsalva manoeuvre

The Valsalva manoeuvre describes the action of forced expiration against a closed glottis. To perform it, patients should be asked to breathe in and then to strain for a few seconds with their breath held. Alternatively, they can be given a 10-mL plastic syringe and asked to 'blow' into the hole to try to push out the plunger from the opposite end. This is impossible to achieve, but in trying to do so the patient effectively performs a Valsalva manoeuvre.

Drug treatments include intravenous adenosine (do not use if the patient has asthma or obstructive airways disease) or intravenous verapamil (not to be used if the patient has recently taken a beta blocker). If the patient is haemodynamically compromised, consider urgent **DC cardioversion** (p. 45) or **overdrive atrial pacing** (Chapter 14).

In the longer term, the arrhythmia does not require prophylactic treatment if episodes are brief and cause few symptoms. Patients can be taught to use the Valsalva manoeuvre. If drug treatment is required, referral to a cardiologist is recommended. Sotalol is often effective as a first-line agent, but radiofrequency ablation via a cardiac catheter can be curative.

Atrial fibrillation in WPW syndrome

AV re-entry tachycardia is not the only arrhythmia seen in WPW syndrome. AF can be precipitated by the re-entry tachycardia. If the patient goes into AF, conduction to the ventricles can occur via either the accessory pathway (which is commonest) or the AV node, or both. Conduction via the accessory pathway can cause a rapid and potentially lethal ventricular rate in response. Drugs that block the AV node (e.g. digoxin, verapamil or adenosine) are therefore hazardous in these patients, as they will increase conduction down the accessory pathway. DC cardioversion is the treatment of choice if the patient is haemodynamically compromised. Recurrent episodes can be treated with drugs that slow conduction in the accessory pathway, such as sotalol, flecainide, disopyramide or amiodarone. Patients resistant to drug therapy should be considered for accessory pathway ablation.

VENTRICULAR TACHYCARDIA

Ventricular tachycardia is a **broad-complex tachycardia**, defined as three or more successive ventricular beats at a heart rate above 120 beats/min. It arises either from a re-entry circuit or from increased automaticity of a specific ventricular focus. Episodes can be self-terminating or sustained (defined as lasting longer than 30 s), and can also degenerate into ventricular fibrillation (VF) (Fig. 3.19).

Characteristic features of VT are:

- ventricular rate above 120/min
- broad QRS complexes.

Sustained VT normally occurs at a heart rate of 150–250/min, but the diagnosis can be difficult. VT can be well tolerated and may not cause haemodynamic disturbance. Do *not* assume, therefore, that just because the patient appears well it is not VT. Help with distinguishing VT from arrhythmias with similar ECG appearances is given in the second half of this chapter.

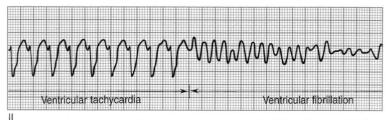

II

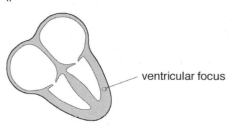

ventricular focus

Fig. 3.19 Ventricular tachycardia (VT) and ventricular fibrillation (VF)

Key points:

- broad-complex tachycardia at a rate of 190/min (VT)

- degenerates into chaotic rhythm (VF)

Table 3.3 Causes of ventricular tachycardia

- Acute myocardial infarction
- Ischaemic heart disease
- Hypertrophic cardiomyopathy
- Dilated cardiomyopathy
- Mitral valve prolapse
- Myocarditis
- Congenital heart disease (repaired or unrepaired)
- Electrolyte disturbance
- Pro-arrhythmic drugs
- Idiopathic

The symptoms of VT can vary from mild palpitations to dizziness, syncope and cardiac arrest. Always look for an underlying treatable cause (Table 3.3).

An episode of VT can be terminated using:

- drugs
- DC cardioversion
- pacing.

Choose the treatment according to the clinical state of the patient. When haemodynamic impairment is present, VT becomes a medical emergency and warrants urgent DC cardioversion (Chapter 17).

ACT QUICKLY

Ventricular tachycardia causing haemodynamic compromise is an emergency. Immediate diagnosis and treatment are required.

Stable patients can be cardioverted medically. Amiodarone is often the first-line agent, but alternatives include lidocaine (lignocaine), flecainide, sotalol and disopyramide. Overdrive right ventricular pacing (Chapter 14) is also effective but may precipitate VF.

Long-term prophylaxis should be discussed with a cardiologist. It usually isn't necessary for VT that occurred within the first 48 h following an acute myocardial infarction. Effective drug treatments include sotalol (particularly when VT is exercise related) and amiodarone. VT related to bradycardia should be treated by pacing. Ablation or surgery can be used to remove a ventricular focus or re-entry circuit identified by electrophysiological testing. Finally, automatic implantable cardioverter defibrillator devices can be implanted to deliver low-energy DC shocks for recurrent episodes of VT (and VF) – see Chapter 14.

 SEEK HELP

The management options for recurrent VT should be discussed with a cardiologist.

ACCELERATED IDIOVENTRICULAR RHYTHM

Accelerated idioventricular rhythm is a slow form of VT, with a heart rate of less than 120 beats/min (Fig. 3.20).

It is usually seen in the setting of an acute myocardial infarction and is benign. No treatment is necessary.

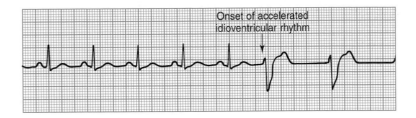

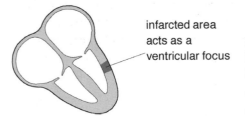

infarcted area
acts as a
ventricular focus

Fig. 3.20 Accelerated
idioventricular rhythm
Key points:
- broad QRS complexes
- heart rate is 60 beats/min

TORSADES DE POINTES

Torsades de pointes is an unusual variant of polymorphic VT
that is associated with a long QT interval (p. 198). Its name
derives from the characteristic undulating pattern on the ECG,
with a variation in the direction of the QRS axis (Fig. 3.21).

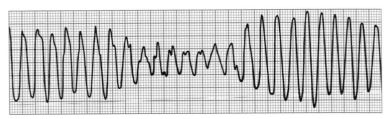

II

Fig. 3.21 Torsades de pointes
Key points: • broad-complex tachycardia (rate is 270/min)
• variation in QRS axis

It can occur with certain anti-arrhythmic drug treatments,
electrolyte abnormalities and hereditary syndromes (see
Chapter 11). As it carries a risk of precipitating VF, urgent
assessment is warranted, with referral to a cardiologist if

necessary. Any causative drugs need to be identified and withdrawn, and electrolyte abnormalities corrected.

In an emergency, torsades de pointes can be treated with beta blockers, magnesium and temporary pacing, which increases the heart rate and thereby shortens the QT interval. In the congenital long QT syndromes, beta blockers or left cervical sympathectomy are indicated to interrupt the sympathetic supply to the heart. An implantable cardiac defibrillator may be required if the patient is judged to be at high risk of sudden cardiac death.

 SEEK HELP

Torsades de pointes can cause VF. Urgent referral to a cardiologist is recommended.

VENTRICULAR FIBRILLATION

Untreated VF is a rapidly fatal arrhythmia. It therefore requires immediate diagnosis and treatment. Turn to Chapter 17 to find the emergency management algorithm for this arrhythmia.

VF is most commonly seen in the setting of an acute myocardial infarction. Always check for electrolyte or acid–base abnormalities following an episode of VF. A single episode of **primary** VF (occurring within 48 h of an infarction), once corrected by DC shock, does not require prophylactic treatment.

Recurrent episodes of VF, or **secondary** VF (after 48 h), merit prophylaxis with amiodarone, beta blockers or lignocaine. Long-term prophylaxis is the same as for VT.

 ACT QUICKLY

Ventricular fibrillation is a medical emergency. Immediate diagnosis and treatment are essential.

CONDUCTION DISTURBANCES

The normal conduction of impulses from the SA node to the ventricles is described in Chapter 1. Block can occur at many different points along this route (Fig. 3.22).

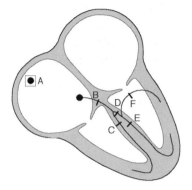

A: Sinoatrial block
B: Atrioventricular block
C: Right bundle branch block
D: Left bundle branch block
E: Left posterior fascicular hemiblock
F: Left anterior fascicular hemiblock

Fig. 3.22 Regions where conduction blocks can occur

In **sinoatrial block**, the SA node depolarizes as normal, but the impulse fails to reach the atria. A P wave fails to appear in the expected place, but the next one usually appears exactly on time. An example is shown in Fig. 3.7.

Atrioventricular block (Chapter 6) is of three degrees of severity. First-degree AV block simply lengthens the PR interval by delaying conduction through the AV node. In second-degree AV block, some atrial impulses fail to be conducted to the ventricles. In third-degree AV block, there is no conduction between atria and ventricles.

Further down the conducting system, **bundle branch block** can affect either the left or right bundle branch. Sometimes only one of the two fascicles of the left bundle branch is affected. Any permutation of these is possible, and block of both bundle branches together is equivalent to third-degree AV block, as no impulses will reach the ventricular myocardium. Bundle branch block is discussed on p. 143, and fascicular block on pp. 90 and 96.

Conduction disturbances are not always a consistent feature of the ECG. They can be rate dependent, only appearing at high heart rates when compromised regions of the conducting system fail to keep pace with the conduction of impulses. The development of bundle branch block during a supraventricular tachycardia (SVT), for example, can give it the appearance of VT (p. 73).

Conduction disturbances are important to recognize, not only because of their effects on the appearance of the ECG but also because escape rhythms can appear when there is complete block of normal conduction.

ESCAPE RHYTHMS

Escape rhythms are a form of 'safety net' for the heart. Without escape rhythms, complete failure of impulse generation or conduction at any time would lead to ventricular asystole and death. Instead, the heart has a number of subsidiary pacemakers that can take over if normal impulse generation or conduction fails.

The subsidiary pacemakers are located in the AV junction and the ventricular myocardium. If the AV junction fails to receive impulses, as a result of SA arrest or block, or even during severe sinus bradycardia, it will take over as the cardiac pacemaker. The QRS complex(es) generated will have the same morphology as normal, but at a slower rate of around 40–60 beats/min (Fig. 3.23).

The AV junctional pacemaker will continue until it again starts to be inhibited by impulses from the SA node. If the AV junctional pacemaker fails, or its impulses are blocked, a ventricular pacemaker will take over. Its rhythm is even slower, at 15–40 beats/min, and the QRS complexes will be broad (Fig. 3.24).

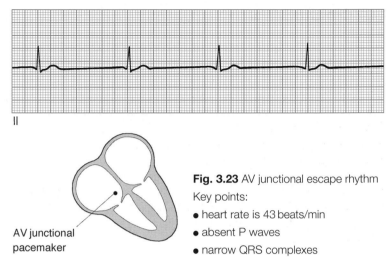

Fig. 3.23 AV junctional escape rhythm

Key points:

- heart rate is 43 beats/min
- absent P waves
- narrow QRS complexes

AV junctional pacemaker

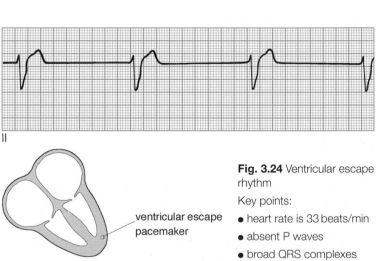

Fig. 3.24 Ventricular escape rhythm

Key points:

- heart rate is 33 beats/min
- absent P waves
- broad QRS complexes

ventricular escape pacemaker

Because escape rhythms exist as a safety net, they must *not* be suppressed. Instead, you must identify why the escape rhythm has arisen (i.e. why normal impulse generation has failed or been blocked) and correct that underlying problem. This will usually require a pacemaker, and should be discussed with a cardiologist.

ECTOPIC BEATS

In contrast to the QRS complexes of escape rhythms, which appear *later* than expected, ectopic beats appear *earlier* than expected. They can arise from any region of the heart, but are normally classified into atrial, AV junctional and ventricular ectopics. Ectopic beats are also called **extrasystoles** and **premature beats**.

Atrial ectopics are identified by a P wave that appears earlier than expected and has an abnormal shape (Fig. 3.25). Although atrial ectopic beats will usually be conducted to the ventricles and give rise to a QRS complex, occasionally they may encounter a refractory AV node and fail to be conducted.

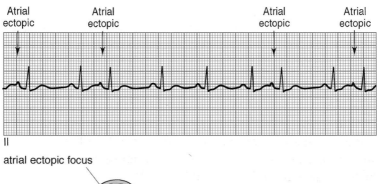

Fig. 3.25 Atrial ectopic beats
Key points:
- P waves earlier than expected
- P wave abnormally shaped

AV junctional ectopics will activate the ventricles, giving rise to a QRS complex earlier than expected (Fig. 3.26). They may also retrogradely activate the atria to cause an inverted P wave. Whether the P wave occurs before, during or after the

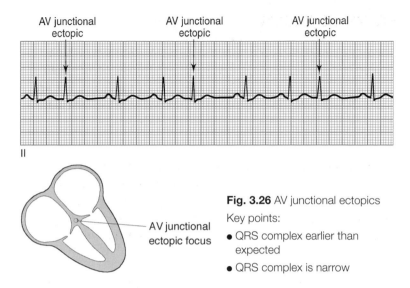

AV junctional ectopic   AV junctional ectopic   AV junctional ectopic

II

AV junctional ectopic focus

Fig. 3.26 AV junctional ectopics

Key points:
- QRS complex earlier than expected
- QRS complex is narrow

QRS complex simply depends upon whether the electrical impulse reaches the atria or ventricles first.

Ventricular ectopics give rise to broad QRS complexes. Occasionally, they will be followed by inverted P waves if the atria are activated by retrograde conduction. If retrograde conduction does not occur, there will usually be a full compensatory pause before the next normal beat because the SA node will not be 'reset' (Fig. 3.27).

Ventricular ectopics can occur at the same time as the T wave of the preceding beat. In the setting of an acute myocardial infarction, such 'R on T' ectopics can trigger ventricular arrhythmias.

Ventricular ectopics can be frequent. When one ectopic follows every normal beat, the term 'bigeminy' is used (Fig. 3.28).

Despite the fact that some ventricular ectopics can precipitate fatal arrhythmias, routine treatment with anti-arrhythmic drugs has not been shown to decrease mortality. Some patients may be significantly troubled by symptoms caused by

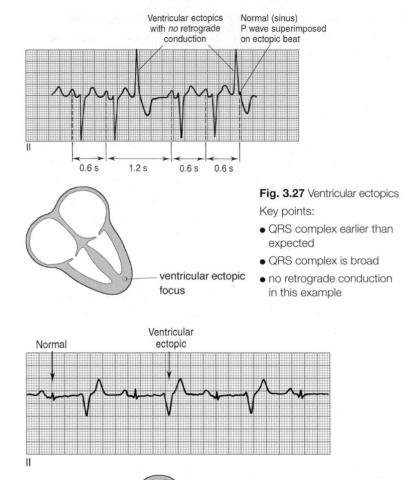

Ventricular ectopics with *no* retrograde conduction

Normal (sinus) P wave superimposed on ectopic beat

II

0.6 s   1.2 s   0.6 s   0.6 s

Fig. 3.27 Ventricular ectopics

Key points:

- QRS complex earlier than expected
- QRS complex is broad
- no retrograde conduction in this example

ventricular ectopic focus

Normal   Ventricular ectopic

II

sinoatrial node

ventricular ectopic focus

Fig. 3.28 Bigeminy

Key point: • each normal beat is followed by a ventricular ectopic the ectopic beat, the compensatory pause or the following sinus beat (usually a feeling of 'extra beats', 'missed beats' or 'heavy beats') and will benefit from using an anti-arrhythmic agent.

IDENTIFYING THE CARDIAC RHYTHM

If you have read through the first part of this chapter, you will now have a good idea of the range of normal and abnormal cardiac rhythms, and their causes and treatment, and will be in a good position to identify the cardiac rhythm in any ECG. If you have turned straight to this section, we strongly recommend that you spend some time going through the preceding pages before continuing any further.

In this section, we will teach you a routine to guide you towards the correct diagnosis of any rhythm disorder. Before doing this, we will repeat the warning with which we started this chapter.

 SEEK HELP

If in doubt about a patient's cardiac rhythm, do not hesitate to seek the advice of a cardiologist.

We trust that the advice given here will be sufficient to keep you out of trouble when trying to identify the cardiac rhythm in an emergency. However, the recognition of some arrhythmias can be difficult, even for the specialist, and if you are at all uncertain about the diagnosis, it is important that you seek expert help at the earliest opportunity.

When you analyse the cardiac rhythm, always keep in mind the two questions that you are trying to answer:

● Where does the impulse arise from?
  – SA node

- atria
- AV junction
- ventricles
● How is the impulse conducted?
- normal conduction
- accelerated conduction (e.g. WPW syndrome)
- blocked conduction.

We will help you to narrow down the possible diagnoses with the following questions.

● What electrical activity is present?
● What is the ventricular rate?
● Is the ventricular rhythm regular or irregular?
● Is the QRS complex width normal or broad?
● Is atrial activity present?
● How are atrial activity and ventricular activity related?

A similar approach to the ECG is used by the Resuscitation Council (UK) to train healthcare professionals in rhythm recognition. Attending a course in Advanced Life Support (ALS) is an excellent way to improve your skills in cardiac rhythm recognition and, of course, in learning how to provide advanced life support. Contact details for the Resuscitation Council (UK) are provided in the further reading section at the end of this book. If you live outside the UK, you should approach your local provider of ALS training for advice.

What electrical activity is present?

Begin by looking at the ECG as a whole for the presence of electrical activity. If there is none, assess the patient (do they have a pulse?), the electrodes (has something become disconnected?) and the gain setting (is the gain setting on the monitor too low?).

If the patient is pulseless with no electrical activity evident on the ECG, they are in **asystole** and appropriate emergency action must be taken – see Chapter 17 for more details. Beware of diagnosing asystole in the presence of a completely

flat ECG trace – there is usually some baseline drift present.
A completely flat line usually means an electrode has become
disconnected – check the electrodes (and, of course, the
patient) carefully when making your diagnosis.

P waves may appear on their own (for a short time) after the
onset of ventricular asystole. The presence of 'P waves only' on
the ECG is important to recognize, as the patient may respond
to emergency pacing manoeuvres such as percussion pacing,
transcutaneous pacing or temporary transvenous pacing.

If QRS complexes are present, move on to the next question.

What is the ventricular rate?

Ventricular activity is represented on the ECG by QRS
complexes. The two methods for determining the
ventricular rate are discussed in Chapter 2. Once you have
calculated the ventricular rate, you will be able to classify
the rhythm as:

● bradycardia (<60 beats/min)
● normal (60–100 beats/min)
● tachycardia (>100 beats/min).

Is the ventricular rhythm regular or irregular?

Having determined the ventricular rate, you should determine
its regularity. Look at the spacing between QRS complexes – is
it the same throughout the rhythm strip? Irregularity can be
subtle, so it is useful to measure out the distance between each
QRS complex. One way to do this is to place a piece of paper
alongside the rhythm strip and make a mark on it next to
every QRS complex. By moving the marked paper up and down
along the rhythm strip, you can soon see if the gaps between
each QRS complex stay the same or vary. Once you have
assessed the regularity, you will be able to classify the
ventricular rhythm as:

● regular (equal spacing between QRS complexes)
● irregular (variable spacing between QRS complexes).

Table 3.4 lists the causes of irregular cardiac rhythms.

Table 3.4 Irregular cardiac rhythms

- Atrial fibrillation
- Sinus arrhythmia
- Any supraventricular rhythm with intermittent AV block
- Ectopic beats

If the rhythm is irregular, it is helpful to try to characterize the degree of irregularity. **Atrial fibrillation,** for example, is a totally chaotic rhythm with no discernible pattern to the QRS complexes. **Sinus arrhythmia,** by comparison, shows a cyclical variation in ventricular rate that is not chaotic but has a clear periodicity to it, which coincides with the patient's breathing movements.

In **intermittent AV block,** if an impulse is blocked *en route* to the ventricles as a result of a conduction disturbance, the corresponding QRS complex will fail to appear where expected and the beat will be 'missed' (Fig. 3.29). This is discussed on p. 118. The degree of irregularity will depend upon the nature of the conduction problem – the block of impulses may be predictable, in which case there will be a 'regular irregularity', or unpredictable.

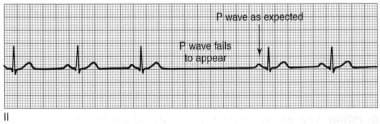

P wave as expected

P wave fails to appear

II

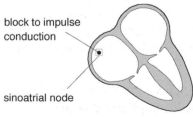

block to impulse conduction

sinoatrial node

Fig. 3.29 Example of a conduction disturbance (sinoatrial block)

Key point:

- P wave fails to appear where expected

Similarly, **ectopic beats** (Fig. 3.30) may occur in a predictable manner or unpredictably, giving rise to regular or irregular irregularities accordingly. In ventricular bigeminy, for example, a ventricular ectopic beat arises after each normal QRS complex, leading to a regular irregularity of the ventricular rhythm (see Fig. 3.28). Ectopic beats are discussed further on p. 60.

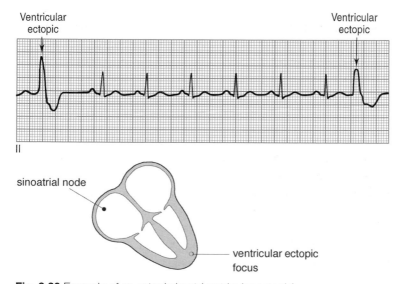

Fig. 3.30 Example of an ectopic beat (ventricular ectopic)
Key point: • ectopic beats appear earlier than expected

Is the QRS complex width normal or broad?

Looking at the width of the QRS complex can provide valuable clues as to the origin of the cardiac rhythm. By answering this question, you will have narrowed down the origin of the impulse to one half of the heart. Ventricular rhythms are generated within the ventricular myocardium; supraventricular rhythms are generated anywhere up to (and including) the AV junction (Fig. 3.31).

Normally, the ventricles are depolarized via the His–Purkinje system, a network of rapidly conducting fibres that run

SUPRAVENTRICULAR

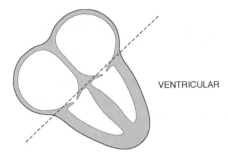

VENTRICULAR

Fig. 3.31 Supraventricular vs ventricular rhythm

Key point:

● supraventricular applies to any structure above the ventricles (and electrically distinct from them)

throughout the ventricular myocardium. As a result, the ventricles are normally completely depolarized within 0.12 s, and the corresponding QRS complex on the ECG is less than 3 small squares wide.

However, if there is a problem with conduction within the ventricles, such as a block of part of the His–Purkinje system (as seen in left or right bundle branch block, RBBB), depolarization has to spread directly from myocyte to myocyte instead. This takes longer, and so the QRS complex becomes wider than 3 small squares. This is also the case if the impulse has arisen within the ventricles (instead of coming via the AV node), as in the case of a ventricular ectopic beat or in VT. If an impulse doesn't pass through the AV node, it can't use the His–Purkinje conduction system. Once again, it must travel from myocyte to myocyte, prolonging the process of depolarization.

This allows us to use the width of the QRS complex to try to determine how the ventricles were depolarized. If the QRS complex is narrow (<3 small squares), the ventricles must have been depolarized by an impulse that came through the AV node – the only way into the His–Purkinje system. The patient is said to have a **supraventricular rhythm** ('arising from above the ventricles').

If the QRS complex is broad (>3 small squares), there are two possible explanations:

1. The impulse may have arisen from within the ventricles and thus been unable to travel via the His–Purkinje system (**ventricular rhythm**).
2. The impulse may have arisen from above the ventricles but not been able to use all the His–Purkinje system because of a conduction problem (**supraventricular rhythm with aberrant conduction**).

This is summarized in Table 3.5.

Table 3.5 Broad-complex vs narrow-complex rhythms

	Broad complex	Narrow complex
Supraventricular rhythm with normal conduction	✗	✓
Supraventricular rhythm with aberrant conduction	✓	✗
Ventricular rhythm	✓	✗

Trying to distinguish between ventricular rhythms and supraventricular rhythms with aberrant conduction can be difficult, particularly if the patient is tachycardic and there is concern that they may have VT. The distinction of VT and SVT discussed specifically on p. 73.

Is atrial activity present?

Atrial electrical activity can take several forms, which can be grouped into four categories:

● P waves (atrial depolarization)
● flutter waves (atrial flutter)
● fibrillation waves (AF)
● unclear activity.

The presence of **P waves** indicates atrial depolarization. This does not mean that the depolarization necessarily started at the SA node, however. P waves will appear during atrial depolarization regardless of where it originated – it is the *orientation* of the P waves that tells you where the depolarization originated (Chapter 5). Upright P waves in lead II suggest that atrial depolarization originated in or near the SA node. Inverted P waves suggest an origin closer to, or within, the AV node (Fig. 3.32).

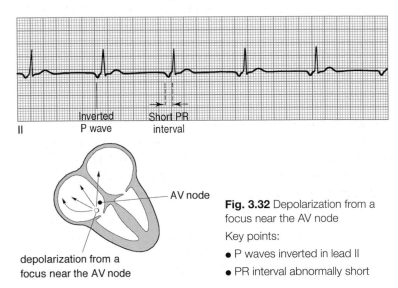

II Inverted P wave Short PR interval

depolarization from a focus near the AV node

AV node

Fig. 3.32 Depolarization from a focus near the AV node

Key points:

- P waves inverted in lead II
- PR interval abnormally short

Flutter waves are seen in atrial flutter at a rate of 300/min, creating a sawtooth baseline of atrial activity (see Fig. 3.11). As discussed earlier, this can be made more readily apparent by manoeuvres that transiently block the AV node.

Fibrillation waves are seen in AF and correspond to random, chaotic atrial impulses occurring at a rate of around 400–600/min (see Fig. 3.13). This leads to a chaotic, low-amplitude baseline of atrial activity.

The nature of the atrial activity may be **unclear**. This may be because P waves are 'hidden' within the QRS complexes, as is often the case during AV nodal re-entry tachycardia. In such cases atrial depolarization is taking place, but its electrical 'signature' on the ECG can't easily be seen because the simultaneous, larger amplitude, QRS complex hides it. Atrial activity may also be absent in, for example, sinus arrest or SA block, in which case the atria may be electrically silent.

How are atrial activity and ventricular activity related?

Having examined the activity of the atria and of the ventricles, the final task is to determine how the two are related. Normally an impulse from the atria goes on to depolarize the ventricles, leading to a 1:1 relationship between P waves and QRS complexes. However, impulses from the atria may sometimes fail to reach the ventricles, or the ventricles may generate their own impulses independent of the atria.

If every QRS complex is associated with a P wave, this indicates that the atria and ventricles are being activated by a common source. This is usually, but not necessarily, the SA node; AV junctional rhythms, for example, will also depolarize both atria and ventricles.

If there are more P waves than QRS complexes, conduction between atria and ventricles is being either partly blocked (with only some impulses getting through) or completely blocked (with the ventricles having developed their own escape rhythm). An example is shown in Fig. 3.33.

More QRS complexes than P waves indicate AV dissociation (p. 122), with the ventricles operating independently of the atria and at a higher rate (Fig. 3.34).

Always bear in mind that the P wave may be difficult or even impossible to discern clearly. Therefore, it can be difficult to say conclusively that atrial activity is absent.

Determining the cardiac rhythm

Using the six questions above, you should be able to diagnose most of the cardiac rhythms described in the first half of this chapter when you next encounter them. Always keep things simple and try to avoid getting side-tracked by unnecessary detail – the diagnosis will often be obvious once you've identified the key features of the ECG. There are a handful of

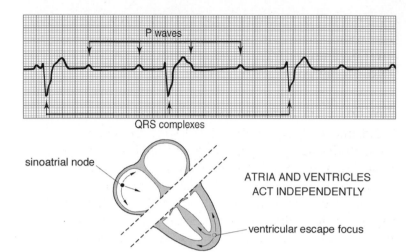

Fig. 3.33 Complete ('third-degree') AV block

Key points: • P wave rate is 75/min

• QRS rate is 33/min

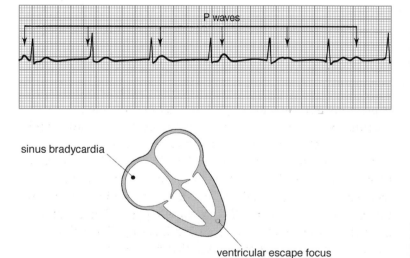

Fig. 3.34 AV dissociation

Key points: • P wave rate 58/min

• QRS rate 65/min

rhythms that you should learn by rote so that you can recognize them without hesitation in an emergency – these are the **cardiac arrest rhythms** (VF, VT, asystole and pulseless electrical activity), which are discussed further in Chapter 17.

How do I distinguish between VT and SVT?

The distinction between VT and SVT with aberrant conduction is not always straightforward, as both can present with a broad-complex tachycardia on the ECG. The distinction is important, as the management of the two conditions is different (although in an emergency both VT and SVT usually respond to DC cardioversion). A good general rule is that *broad-complex tachycardia is always assumed to be VT unless proven otherwise.*

The clinical history may provide a pointer towards the correct diagnosis. A broad-complex tachycardia is more likely to be VT in elderly patients with a history of cardiac disease, and more likely to be SVT with aberrant conduction in young patients with no prior cardiac history. It should not be assumed that patients with VT will always be unwell – some patients tolerate VT remarkably well and can be virtually asymptomatic. Conversely, some patients tolerate SVT very poorly.

A previous ECG may be helpful in determining whether aberrant conduction was present prior to the tachycardia, and whether the QRS morphology has changed. However, it is possible that aberrant conduction has developed in the period between the two ECGs, or that it only appears during the tachycardia. Broad complexes that display a typical left bundle branch block (LBBB) or RBBB morphology (see Chapter 8) are more likely to be due to aberrant conduction; VT usually causes 'atypical' broad complexes that do not have the classical hallmarks of LBBB or RBBB.

A diagnostic feature of VT is the presence of **independent atrial activity**, although it can be found in fewer than half of cases. Independent atrial activity is indicated by:

- independent P wave activity
- fusion beats
- capture beats.

Independent P wave activity is shown by the presence of P waves occurring at a slower rate than the QRS complexes and bearing no relationship to them (Fig. 3.35). It can, however, be difficult or even impossible to discern P waves during VT.

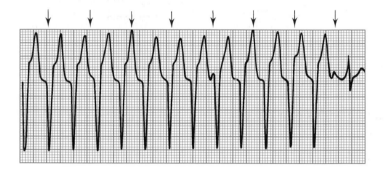

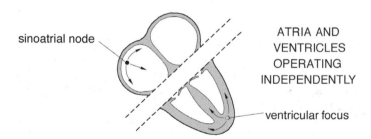

Fig. 3.35 Independent P wave activity

Key points: ● broad-complex tachycardia (VT)

- arrows show independent P waves deforming the QRS complexes
- last beat is a capture beat

Fusion beats appear when the ventricles are activated by an atrial impulse and a ventricular impulse arriving simultaneously (Fig. 3.36).

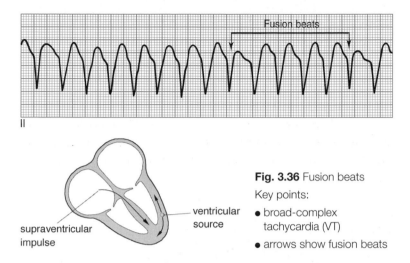

Fig. 3.36 Fusion beats

Key points:
- broad-complex tachycardia (VT)
- arrows show fusion beats

Capture beats occur when an atrial impulse manages to 'capture' the ventricles for a beat, causing a normal QRS complex, which may be preceded by a normal P wave (Fig. 3.37).

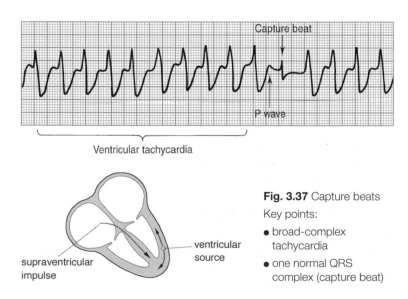

Fig. 3.37 Capture beats

Key points:
- broad-complex tachycardia
- one normal QRS complex (capture beat)

Other clues that suggest that a broad-complex tachycardia is due to VT are:

- QRS duration >0.14 s (3.5 small squares)
- concordance (same QRS direction) in leads V_1–V_6
- a shift in QRS axis of 40° or more (left or right)
- adenosine has no effect.

If the rhythm slows or terminates with manoeuvres that slow or block conduction in the AV node, it is likely to be supraventricular with aberrant conduction.

Supraventricular tachycardia

The term 'supraventricular tachycardia' is frequently misused and this leads to misunderstanding. Literally, it refers to any heart rate over 100 beats/min (tachycardia) that originates above the ventricles (supraventricular). It encompasses many different arrhythmias, including sinus tachycardia, AF, atrial tachycardia and AV re-entry tachycardias. This is the meaning of SVT that has been used in this book. Some people use the term SVT to refer specifically to AV nodal re-entry tachycardias. We recommend that you identify all arrhythmias as specifically as possible, and reserve SVT as a general term for tachycardias that originate above the ventricles.

Summary

When assessing the cardiac rhythm, consider the following:

- SA nodal rhythms
  - sinus rhythm
  - sinus bradycardia
  - sinus tachycardia
  - sinus arrhythmia
  - sick sinus syndrome
- Atrial rhythms
  - atrial tachycardia
  - atrial flutter
  - AF
- AV rhythms
  - AV re-entry tachycardias
- Ventricular rhythms
  - VT
  - accelerated idioventricular rhythm
  - torsades de pointes
  - VF
- Conduction disturbances
- Escape rhythms
- Ectopic beats.

To identify the rhythm, ask the following questions.

1. Where does the impulse arise from?

- SA node
- Atria
- AV junction
- Ventricles.

2. How is the impulse conducted?

- Normal conduction
- Accelerated conduction (e.g. WPW syndrome)
- Blocked conduction.

4

THE AXIS

Working out the cardiac axis causes more confusion than almost any other aspect of ECG assessment. This should not really be the case, as there is no mystery to the cardiac axis and it is usually very straightforward to assess. Indeed, deciding whether the cardiac axis is normal can be summarized in one rule.

A quick rule for assessing the axis

If the QRS complexes are predominantly positive in leads I and II, the cardiac axis is normal.

If you are confident about assessing the axis, you can go straight to the second half of this chapter, where we explain the causes of an abnormal axis. If not, read through the first half of the chapter, where we explain in straightforward terms what the axis represents and how it can be measured.

What does the axis mean?

As we explained in Chapter 1, the flow of electrical current through the heart is fairly uniform, as it normally passes along a well-defined pathway (Fig. 4.1).

In simple terms, the cardiac axis is an indicator of the general direction that the wave of depolarization takes as it flows through the ventricles. If you think just about the general direction of electrical current as it flows through the ventricles, it starts at the 'top right-hand corner' and flows towards the 'bottom left-hand corner' (Fig. 4.2).

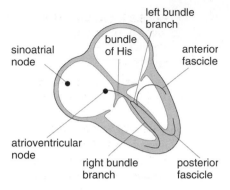

Fig. 4.1 The flow of electrical impulses through the heart

Key points:

• impulses originate in the sinoatrial node

• impulses reach the ventricles via the atrioventricular node

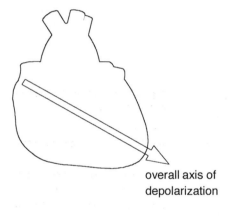

Fig. 4.2 The general direction of flow of electrical current through the heart

Key points:

• flow starts at the 'top right-hand corner'

• flow is towards the 'bottom left-hand corner'

What measurement is used for the axis?

When describing the axis, a more precise terminology is required. The axis is therefore conventionally referred to as the angle, measured in degrees, of the direction of electrical current flowing through the ventricles.

The reference, or zero, point is taken as a horizontal line 'looking' at the heart from the left (Fig. 4.3). For a direction of flow directed below the line, the angle is expressed as a positive number; above the line, as a negative number (Fig. 4.4). Thus, the cardiac axis can be either +1° to +180°, or −1° to −180°.

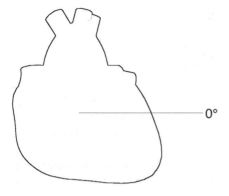

Fig. 4.3 The reference (or 'zero') point for axis measurements

Key points:

● the zero point is a horizontal line looking at the heart from the left

● this is the same as the viewpoint of lead I

● all axis measurements are made relative to this line

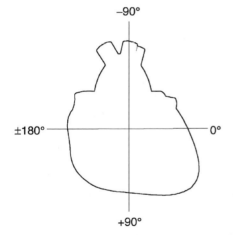

Fig. 4.4 The range of angles of the cardiac axis

Key points:

● anticlockwise measurements are negative

● clockwise measurements are positive

● all measurements are relative to the zero line

You will remember from Chapter 1 that the six limb leads look at the heart sideways from six different viewpoints. The same reference system can be used to describe the angle from which each lead looks at the heart (Fig. 4.5). All the limb leads and their angles are listed in Table 4.1.

Make an effort to remember the viewpoint of each limb lead now, before reading any further. Once you have grasped the concept of each limb lead having a different angle of view of the heart, understanding the cardiac axis will be easy.

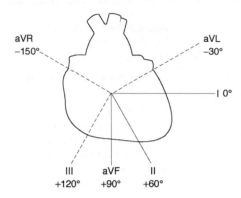

Fig. 4.5 Viewpoints of the six limb leads

Key point:

● each lead looks at the heart from a different angle

Table 4.1 Limb leads and angles of view

Limb lead	Angle at which it views the heart
I	0°
II	+60°
III	+120°
aVR	−150°
aVL	−30°
aVF	+90°

How do I use the limb leads to work out the axis?

The information from the limb leads is used to work out the cardiac axis. Simply remember three principles, all of which we have covered already:

● The axis is the general direction of electrical flow through the heart.
● Each of the limb leads records this electrical flow from a different viewpoint of the heart.
● Electrical flow towards a lead causes a positive deflection, and flow away from a lead causes a negative deflection.

This last rule means that if current flows at right angles to a lead, the ECG complex generated will be isoelectric (the positive and negative deflections cancel each other out). This is illustrated in Fig. 4.6.

Using these principles, consider how lead II records ventricular depolarization. From its point of view, the flow of current in

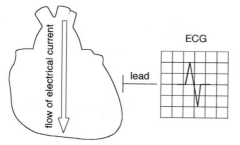

Fig. 4.6 An isoelectric ECG complex

Key point:

- current flow at right angles to a lead causes an isoelectric complex

the ventricles is entirely towards it and the QRS complex is entirely positive (Fig. 4.7). Lead aVL, however, will see the same current at right angles to itself and record an isoelectric QRS complex (Fig. 4.8). Any lead looking from a viewpoint between leads II and aVL will record a complex that becomes increasingly positive the closer it is to lead II (Fig. 4.9).

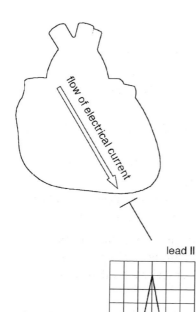

Fig. 4.7 The QRS complex is entirely positive in lead II

Key points:

- flow towards a lead causes a positive deflection
- current flow in the ventricles is towards lead II

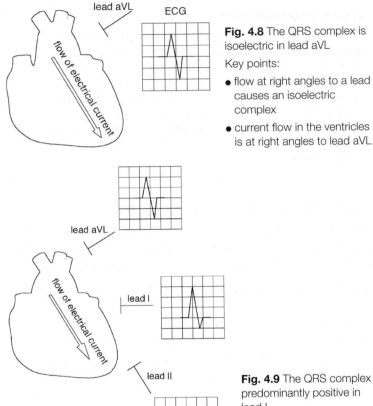

Fig. 4.8 The QRS complex is isoelectric in lead aVL

Key points:

- flow at right angles to a lead causes an isoelectric complex

- current flow in the ventricles is at right angles to lead aVL

Fig. 4.9 The QRS complex is predominantly positive in lead I

Key point:

- lead I lies between leads II and aVL

It should now be fairly clear that you can work out the cardiac axis by examining whether the QRS complexes in the limb leads are predominantly positive or negative.

There are two ways of determining the cardiac axis: one is quick and approximate, the other is precise but detailed.

What is a 'normal' axis?

Unfortunately, there is no universal agreement on what is a normal axis. For the purposes of this book, we consider a normal axis to be anything between −30° and +90°, although we should mention that some cardiologists accept anything up to +120° as normal. This is because there is no definitive dividing line between normality and abnormality. The most sensible approach is to consider that the likelihood of a patient having an underlying abnormality increases as the axis increases from +90° to +120°.

A quick way to work out the cardiac axis

This technique enables you to decide within seconds whether the axis is normal or abnormal. To decide if the axis is normal, you need only look at two of the limb leads: I and II.

If the QRS complex in **lead I** is predominantly positive, this indicates that the axis lies anywhere between −90° and +90° (Fig. 4.10). An axis at *exactly* −90° or +90° would cause a precisely isoelectric QRS complex in lead I. Thus, a predominantly positive QRS complex in lead I rules out right axis deviation (an axis beyond +90°), but does not exclude left axis deviation (an axis beyond −30°).

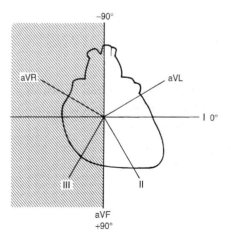

Fig. 4.10 A predominantly positive QRS in lead I puts the axis between −90° and +90°

Key point:

- a predominantly positive QRS in lead I excludes right axis deviation

If the QRS complex in **lead II** is predominantly positive, this indicates that the axis lies anywhere between $-30°$ and $+150°$ (Fig. 4.11). An axis at *exactly* $-30°$ or $+150°$ would cause a precisely isoelectric QRS complex in lead II. Thus, a predominantly positive QRS complex in lead II rules out left axis deviation (an axis beyond $-30°$), but does not exclude right axis deviation (an axis beyond $+90°$).

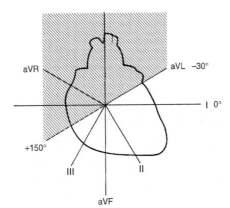

Fig. 4.11 A predominantly positive QRS in lead II puts the axis between $-30°$ and $+150°$

Key point:

● a predominantly positive QRS in lead II excludes left axis deviation

However, by looking at whether the QRS complex is positive or negative in both these leads, it is possible to say immediately whether the axis is normal, or whether there is left or right axis deviation:

● A predominantly positive QRS complex in both leads I and II means the **axis is normal**.
● A predominantly positive QRS complex in lead I and a predominantly negative QRS complex in lead II mean there is **left axis deviation**.
● A predominantly negative QRS complex in lead I and a predominantly positive QRS complex in lead II mean there is **right axis deviation**.

These rules are summarized in Table 4.2.

Table 4.2 Working out the cardiac axis

Lead I	Lead II	Cardiac axis
Positive QRS	Positive QRS	Normal axis
Positive QRS	Negative QRS	Left axis deviation
Negative QRS	Positive QRS	Right axis deviation

When you assess the cardiac axis you should therefore ask the following questions:

● Is there left axis deviation?
● Is there right axis deviation?

The causes of these abnormalities, with guidance on their management, are discussed in the second half of this chapter.

A more precise way to calculate the cardiac axis

For most practical purposes, it is not necessary to determine precisely the axis of the heart – it is sufficient to know simply whether the axis is normal or abnormal. Calculating the axis precisely is not difficult but does take a little time – this section explains how.

The method relies upon the use of vectors and knowledge of how to calculate angles in right-angled triangles. Begin by finding two leads that look at the heart at right angles to each other, for example leads I and aVF (Fig. 4.12).

Look at the QRS complexes in these leads, and work out their overall sizes and polarities by subtracting the depth of the S wave from the height of the R wave (Fig. 4.13). The polarity (positive or negative) tells you whether the impulse is moving towards or away from the lead. The overall size tells you how much of the electricity is flowing in that direction. Using this information, you can construct a vector diagram (Fig. 4.14).

Thus, by combining the information from the two leads, you can use a pocket calculator to work out the angle at which the current is flowing (i.e. the cardiac axis).

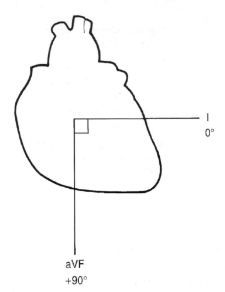

Fig. 4.12 Leads I and aVF

Key point:

• leads I and aVF are at right angles to each other

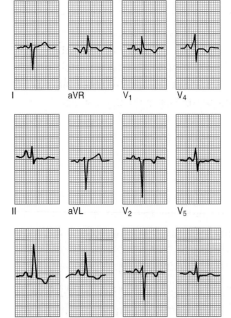

Fig. 4.13 Overall size and polarity of QRS complexes in leads I and aVF

Key points:

• overall QRS 'height' is −8 mm in lead I

• overall QRS 'height' is +9 mm in lead aVF

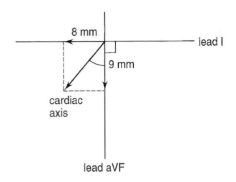

Fig. 4.14 Constructing a vector diagram

Key points:

- draw arrows to represent the QRS 'heights' from Fig. 4.13

- the cardiac axis lies between the arrows

- use sine, cosine or tangent to work out the exact angle of the axis

---

Remember

- sine of an angle = opposite edge/hypotenuse
- cosine of an angle = adjacent edge/hypotenuse
- tangent of an angle = opposite edge/adjacent edge.

Thus, we finally arrive at an angle in degrees (Fig. 4.15). Do not forget that the cardiac axis is measured relative to lead I, and to add or subtract units of 90° accordingly. The axis in this patient is therefore +132°, and he or she has (by our definition) right axis deviation. We recommend that you practise this technique to become fully familiar with it.

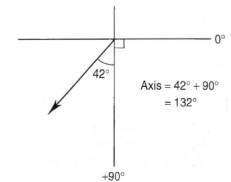

Axis = 42° + 90°
    = 132°

Fig. 4.15 Working out the cardiac axis

Key point:

- do not forget to add or subtract units of 90° according to which quadrant the axis lies in

---

P and T wave axes

So far, we have concentrated on the axis of depolarization as it flows through the ventricles, and this is generally referred to as the cardiac axis. However, it is also possible to work out an axis for atrial depolarization (by applying the vector analysis we have described to P waves) and for ventricular repolarization (using T waves). These measurements are seldom necessary, except where a more detailed analysis of the ECG is required.

IS THERE LEFT AXIS DEVIATION?

Left axis deviation is present when the cardiac axis lies beyond $-30°$. This sometimes occurs in normal individuals, but more often indicates one of the following:

- left anterior hemiblock
- Wolff–Parkinson–White (WPW) syndrome
- inferior myocardial infarction
- ventricular tachycardia.

These are discussed on the following pages.

Left ventricular hypertrophy can cause left axis deviation but *not* as a result of increased muscle mass (unlike right ventricular hypertrophy). Instead, it results from left anterior hemiblock caused by fibrosis. Contrary to some textbooks, neither obesity nor pregnancy causes left axis deviation (although obesity can cause a leftward shift with the axis staying within normal limits).

Left anterior hemiblock

In Chapter 1, we describe how electrical impulses are conducted within the interventricular septum in the left and right bundle branches, and that the left bundle branch divides into anterior and posterior fascicles (see Fig. 1.16). Either (or both) of these fascicles can be blocked. Block of the left anterior fascicle is called left anterior hemiblock, and is the commonest cause of left axis deviation (Fig. 4.16).

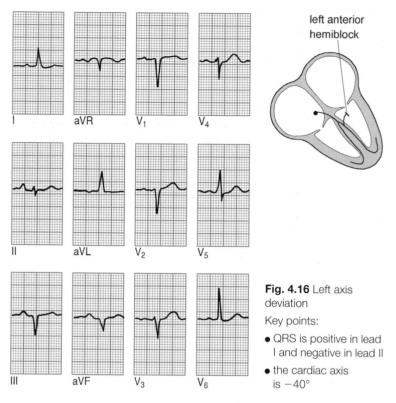

left anterior
hemiblock

Fig. 4.16 Left axis
deviation

Key points:

● QRS is positive in lead
  I and negative in lead II

● the cardiac axis
  is −40°

Left anterior hemiblock can occur as a result of fibrosis of
the conducting system (of any cause), or from myocardial
infarction. On its own, it is not thought to carry any prognostic
significance. However, left anterior hemiblock in combination
with right bundle branch block (p. 144) means that two of the
three main conducting pathways to the ventricles are blocked.
This is termed **bifascicular block** (Fig. 4.17).

Block of the conducting pathways can occur in any
combination. A block of both fascicles is the equivalent of
left bundle branch block. Block of the right bundle branch
and either fascicle is bifascicular block. If bifascicular block
is combined with first-degree AV block (long PR interval),
this is called **trifascicular block** (Fig. 4.18). Block of the
right bundle branch and both fascicles leaves no route for

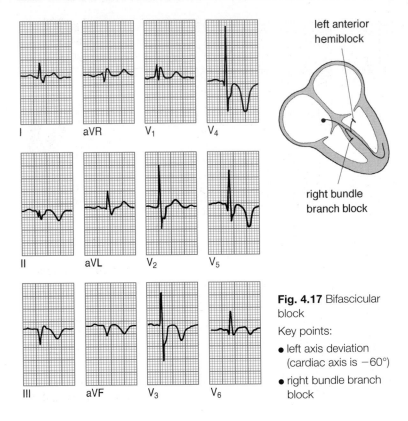

Fig. 4.17 Bifascicular block

Key points:

- left axis deviation (cardiac axis is −60°)
- right bundle branch block

impulses to reach the ventricles, and this is the equivalent of third-degree ('complete') AV block.

Bifascicular block in a patient with syncopal episodes is often sufficient indication for a permanent pacemaker, even if higher degrees of block have not been documented. Referral of these patients to a cardiologist is therefore recommended. *Asymptomatic* bifascicular block, or even trifascicular block, is not necessarily an indication for pacing – discuss with a cardiologist if in doubt.

 SEEK HELP

Bifascicular block with syncope usually requires pacing. Referral to a cardiologist is recommended.

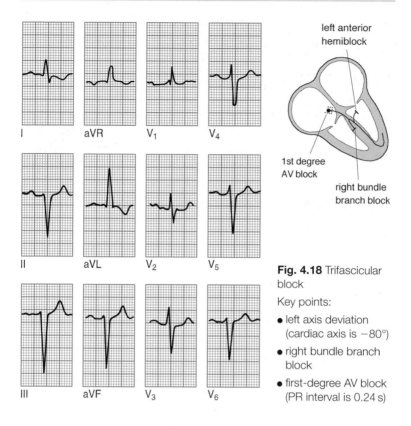

I   aVR   V₁   V₄

II   aVL   V₂   V₅

III   aVF   V₃   V₆

left anterior
hemiblock

1st degree
AV block

right bundle
branch block

Fig. 4.18 Trifascicular block

Key points:

- left axis deviation (cardiac axis is −80°)
- right bundle branch block
- first-degree AV block (PR interval is 0.24 s)

Wolff–Parkinson–White syndrome

Patients with WPW syndrome have an accessory pathway that bypasses the atrioventricular (AV) node and bundle of His to connect the atria directly to the ventricles. If this pathway lies between the atria and ventricles on the right side of the heart, patients may have left axis deviation in addition to the other ECG appearances of WPW syndrome. WPW syndrome is discussed on p. 111.

Inferior myocardial infarction

Left axis deviation may be a feature of myocardial infarction affecting the inferior aspect of the heart (the cardiac axis is directed away from infarcted areas). The diagnosis will usually be apparent from the presentation and other ECG findings.

For more information on the diagnosis and treatment of acute myocardial infarction, turn to Chapter 9.

Ventricular tachycardia (with LV apical focus)

When ventricular tachycardia arises from a focus in the left ventricle, the wave of depolarization spreads out through the rest of the myocardium from that point, resulting in left axis deviation. The diagnosis and treatment of ventricular tachycardia are discussed on p. 52.

IS THERE RIGHT AXIS DEVIATION?

Right axis deviation is present when the cardiac axis lies beyond +90°. This sometimes occurs in normal individuals, but more often indicates one of the following:

● right ventricular hypertrophy
● WPW syndrome
● anterolateral myocardial infarction
● dextrocardia
● left posterior hemiblock.

These are discussed on the following pages.

Right ventricular hypertrophy

Right ventricular hypertrophy is the commonest cause of right axis deviation (Fig. 4.19).

Other ECG evidence of right ventricular hypertrophy includes:

● dominant R wave in lead V_1
● deep S waves in leads V_5 and V_6
● right bundle branch block.

For more information on the causes of right ventricular hypertrophy, turn to p. 135.

Wolff–Parkinson–White syndrome

As with right-sided accessory pathways and left axis deviation, patients with WPW syndrome who have a left-sided accessory

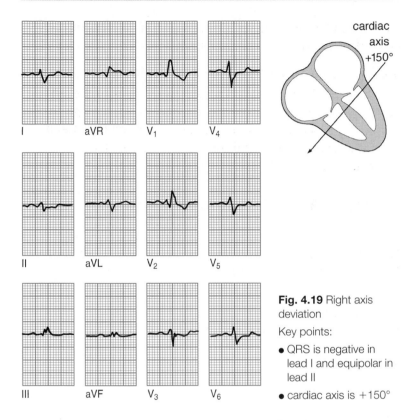

Fig. 4.19 Right axis deviation

Key points:

- QRS is negative in lead I and equipolar in lead II
- cardiac axis is +150°

pathway may have right axis deviation in addition to the other ECG appearances of WPW syndrome. WPW syndrome is discussed in more detail on p. 111.

Anterolateral myocardial infarction

The cardiac axis is directed away from infarcted areas. Thus, right axis deviation may be a feature of anterolateral myocardial infarction. The diagnosis will usually be apparent from the presentation and other ECG findings. For more information on the diagnosis and treatment of acute myocardial infarction, turn to Chapter 9.

Dextrocardia

Right axis deviation is a feature of dextrocardia (in which the heart lies on the right side of the chest instead of the left), but the most obvious abnormality is that all the chest leads have 'right ventricular' QRS complexes (see Fig. 8.5). Dextrocardia is discussed in more detail on p. 139.

Left posterior hemiblock

Unlike left anterior hemiblock, left posterior hemiblock is extremely rare. It is identified in approximately only 1 in every 10 000 ECGs. It is therefore extremely important that if you identify right axis deviation on an ECG, you rule out other causes (in particular, right ventricular hypertrophy) before diagnosing left posterior hemiblock. The causes and management of left posterior hemiblock are the same as for left anterior hemiblock (p. 90).

Summary

To assess the cardiac axis, ask the following questions:

1. Is there left axis deviation?

If 'yes', consider:
- left anterior hemiblock
- WPW syndrome
- inferior myocardial infarction
- ventricular tachycardia (with left ventricular apical focus).

2. Is there right axis deviation?

If 'yes', consider:
- right ventricular hypertrophy
- WPW syndrome
- anterolateral myocardial infarction
- dextrocardia
- left posterior hemiblock.

5

THE P WAVE

After determining the heart rate, rhythm and axis, you should examine each wave of the ECG in turn, beginning with the P wave. You may already have noticed abnormal P waves while assessing the cardiac rhythm, but in this chapter we tell you how to examine the P wave in more detail and what abnormalities to look out for.

As you examine the P wave in each lead, the questions to ask are:

- Are any P waves absent?
- Are any P waves inverted?
- Are any P waves too tall?
- Are any P waves too wide?

In this chapter, we help you to answer these questions and to interpret any abnormalities you may find.

The origin of the P wave

You will recall from Chapter 1 that the P wave represents atrial depolarization. It does not, as some people mistakenly believe, represent sinoatrial (SA) node depolarization; it is possible to have P waves without SA node depolarization (e.g. atrial ectopics), or SA node depolarization without P waves (SA block).

ARE ANY P WAVES ABSENT?

The SA node is normally a very regular and dependable natural pacemaker. Atrial depolarization (and thus P wave formation) is therefore normally so regular that it is easy to predict when the next P wave is going to appear (Fig. 5.1).

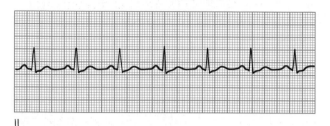

II

sinoatrial node

Fig. 5.1 Sinus rhythm
Key points:
- regular P waves
- it is easy to predict when the next P wave will appear

The only normal circumstance in which the P wave rate is variable is sinus arrhythmia, which is usually only seen in patients below the age of 40 years. Sinus arrhythmia is discussed on p. 35.

In this section, we tell you what diagnoses to consider if you find that P waves are absent. By this, we mean that they can be either:

- completely absent (no P waves on the whole ECG), or
- intermittently absent (some P waves do not appear where expected).

P waves are completely absent

There are two reasons why P waves may be absent from the ECG. The first is that there is no coordinated atrial activity so that P waves are not being formed. The second is that P waves *are* present, but are just not obvious.

A lack of coordinated atrial activity occurs in **atrial fibrillation**, and this is the commonest reason for P waves to be truly absent from the ECG (Fig. 5.2). Instead of P waves, the chaotic atrial activity produces low-amplitude oscillations (fibrillation or 'f' waves) on the ECG. Atrial fibrillation can be recognized by the absence of P waves and the erratic formation of QRS complexes. Atrial fibrillation is discussed on p. 43.

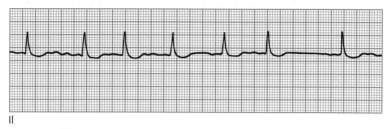

II

multi atrial foci

Fig. 5.2 Atrial fibrillation

Key points:

- absent P waves
- erratic ('irregularly irregular') QRS rhythm

P waves will also be completely absent if there is a prolonged period of **sinus arrest** or **sinoatrial block** (Fig. 5.3). In these conditions, atrial activation does not occur because the SA node either fails to depolarize (sinus arrest) or fails to transmit the depolarization to the atria (SA block). Either condition *can* cause ventricular asystole, but more commonly an escape rhythm takes over (p. 58). See p. 36 for more information on sinus arrest and SA block.

Absent P waves are also one of the possible ECG manifestations of **hyperkalaemia** (p. 178). If this is a possibility, look for associated ECG abnormalities and check the patient's plasma potassium level urgently.

It is very common for P waves to be present but not immediately obvious. Search the ECG carefully for evidence of P waves before concluding that they are absent, as P waves

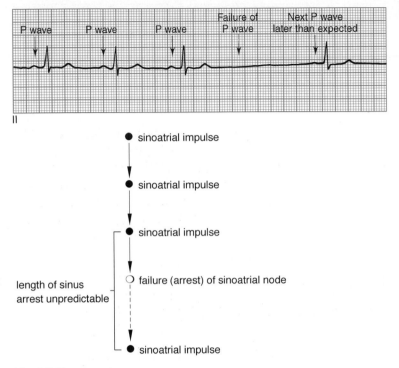

Fig. 5.3 Sinus arrest

Key points:
- failure of P wave to appear when predicted
- the next P wave appears later than expected
- the sinoatrial 'clock' has therefore reset

will often be hidden by any **rapid tachycardia**. Figure 5.4 shows an atrioventricular (AV) junctional tachycardia with a heart rate of 130 beats/min. At first glance, the P waves appear to be absent. On closer inspection, they can just be seen buried within the ST segments.

Even in sinus tachycardia, at high heart rates the P wave may start to overlap with the T wave of the previous beat, making it hard to identify (Fig. 5.5).

At very high atrial rates, such as in atrial flutter, P waves may not be apparent because they become distorted. In atrial flutter,

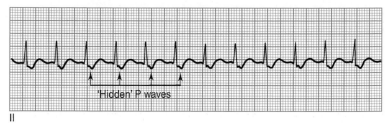

'Hidden' P waves

II

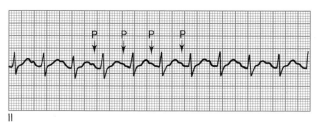

sinoatrial node

Fig. 5.4 AV junctional tachycardia

Key points:

- heart rate is 130 beats/min
- narrow QRS complexes
- P waves 'hidden' within the ST segments

P P P P

II

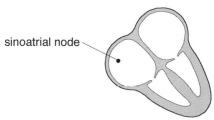

sinoatrial node

Fig. 5.5 Sinus tachycardia

Key points:

- heart rate is 130 beats/min
- narrow QRS complexes
- P waves 'hidden' within the previous T waves

the atria usually depolarize around 300 times/min. The P waves generated by this rapid activity are called flutter waves, and have a 'sawtooth' appearance. Atrial flutter is discussed on p. 40.

In ventricular tachycardia, retrograde (backward) conduction up through the AV node may cause each ventricular complex to be *followed* by a P wave which may not be immediately obvious and which also, incidentally, will be inverted. Even more importantly, *independent* atrial activity can occur during ventricular tachycardia, and the P waves can be buried anywhere within the QRS complexes (see Fig. 3.35). Evidence of independent atrial activity is a very useful clue in the differentiation of ventricular and supraventricular tachycardias.

More information about all of these cardiac rhythms can be found in Chapter 3.

P waves are intermittently absent

The SA node is usually an extremely reliable natural pacemaker. The occasional absence of a P wave on an ECG indicates that the SA node has either failed to generate an impulse (sinus arrest) or failed to conduct the impulse to the surrounding atrial tissue (SA block).

For examples of both these conditions, together with guidance on how to distinguish them, turn to p. 36.

ARE ANY P WAVES INVERTED?

The P wave is usually upright in all leads except aVR, which 'looks' at the atria from roughly the patient's right shoulder and so detects the wave of atrial depolarization moving away from it (see Fig. 1.8). The P wave may sometimes be inverted in lead V_1 also, although it is more usually biphasic in that lead (Fig. 5.6).

Whenever you see an inverted P wave, ask yourself:

● Were the electrodes correctly positioned?

Abnormal P wave inversion can indicate either of the following:

● dextrocardia
● abnormal atrial depolarization.

Dextrocardia is discussed on p. 139. Abnormal atrial depolarization is explained below.

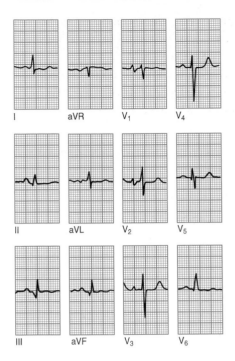

I   aVR   V₁   V₄

II   aVL   V₂   V₅

III   aVF   V₃   V₆

Fig. 5.6 Biphasic P wave
Key point:
● P wave biphasic in lead V₁ (and V₂)

Abnormal atrial depolarization

The wave of depolarization normally spreads through the atria from the SA node to the AV node. If atrial depolarization is initiated from within, near or through the AV node, the wave will travel in the opposite (retrograde) direction through the atria. From the 'viewpoints' of most of the ECG electrodes, this wave will be moving *away from* rather than towards them, and *inverted* P waves will be produced (Fig. 5.7).

Many abnormal sources of atrial activation can thus cause retrograde depolarization and inverted P waves, including:

● atrial ectopics
● AV junctional rhythms
● ventricular tachycardia (retrogradely conducted)
● ventricular ectopics (retrogradely conducted).

A discussion of how to identify and manage all of these rhythms can be found in Chapter 3.

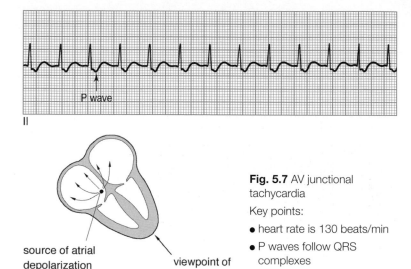

source of atrial
depolarization

viewpoint of
lead II

Fig. 5.7 AV junctional
tachycardia

Key points:

- heart rate is 130 beats/min
- P waves follow QRS
  complexes
- P waves inverted in lead II

ARE ANY P WAVES TOO TALL?

Tall, peaked P waves indicate right atrial enlargement.
The abnormality is sometimes referred to as 'P pulmonale',
because right atrial enlargement is often secondary to
pulmonary disorders. There is no clear 'normal range' for P
wave height, but any P wave over 2.5 mm (2.5 small squares)
in height should arouse suspicion. An example is shown in
Fig. 5.8.

If the P waves appear unusually tall, assess your
patient for any of the causes of right atrial enlargement
(Table 5.1).

Abnormally tall P waves should draw attention to the
possibility of an underlying disorder that may require further
investigation. In addition to a thorough patient history and
examination, a chest X-ray (to assess cardiac dimensions and
lung fields) and an echocardiogram (to assess valvular
disorders and estimate pulmonary artery pressure) may be
helpful.

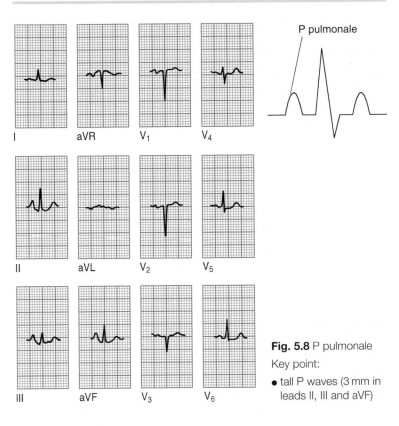

Fig. 5.8 P pulmonale

Key point:

• tall P waves (3 mm in leads II, III and aVF)

Table 5.1 Causes of right atrial enlargement

- Primary pulmonary hypertension
- Secondary pulmonary hypertension
    - chronic bronchitis
    - emphysema
    - massive pulmonary embolism
- Pulmonary stenosis
- Tricuspid stenosis

ARE ANY P WAVES TOO WIDE?

Any P waves that are abnormally wide (>0.08 s, or 2 small squares across) and bifid should raise the suspicion of left atrial enlargement. This is usually a result of mitral valve disease, and consequently the broad, bifid P waves are known as 'P mitrale' (Fig. 5.9).

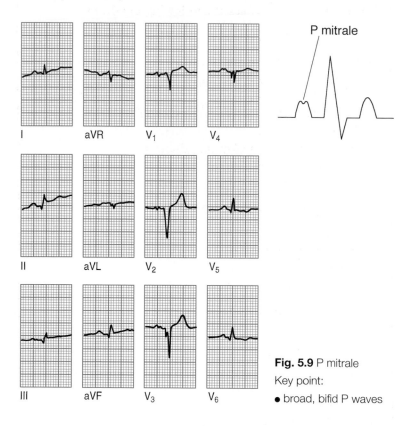

Fig. 5.9 P mitrale
Key point:
- broad, bifid P waves

The P wave becomes broad because the enlarged left atrium takes longer than normal to depolarize. As with P pulmonale, P mitrale does not require treatment in its own right, but should alert you to a possible underlying problem. This is often mitral valve disease, but left atrial enlargement can also accompany left ventricular hypertrophy (e.g. secondary to hypertension, aortic valve disease and hypertrophic cardiomyopathy). A chest X-ray and an echocardiogram may be helpful following a patient history and examination.

Summary

To assess the P wave, ask the following questions:

1. Are any P waves absent?

If 'yes', consider:
- P waves are completely absent
  - atrial fibrillation
  - sinus arrest or SA block (prolonged)
  - hyperkalaemia
- P waves are present but not obvious
- P waves are intermittently absent
  - sinus arrest or SA block (intermittent).

2. Are any P waves inverted?

If 'yes', consider:
- electrode misplacement
- dextrocardia
- retrograde atrial depolarization.

3. Are any P waves too tall?

If 'yes', consider:
- right atrial enlargement.

4. Are any P waves too wide?

If 'yes', consider:
- left atrial enlargement.

6

THE PR INTERVAL

O nce the sinus node has generated an electrical stimulus, this must be transmitted through the atria, atrioventricular (AV) node and bundle of His to reach the ventricles and bring about cardiac contraction. The time delay while this occurs is mainly taken up by the passage of the electrical impulse through the AV node, which acts as a regulator of conduction. This corresponds to the PR interval on the ECG (Fig. 6.1).

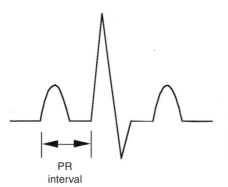

PR
interval

Fig. 6.1 The PR interval
Key point:

- PR interval is measured from the start of the P wave to the start of the R wave

The PR interval has precise time limits. In health, this interval is:

- no less than 0.12 s (3 small squares) long
- no more than 0.2 s (5 small squares) long
- consistent in length.

Make sure you check the duration of as many consecutive PR intervals as you can and ask the following questions:

- Is the PR interval less than 0.12 s long?
- Is the PR interval more than 0.2 s long?
- Does the PR interval vary or can it not be measured?

This chapter will help you to answer these questions and to reach a diagnosis if you find any abnormalities.

IS THE PR INTERVAL LESS THAN 0.12 SECONDS LONG?

A PR interval of less than 0.12 s (3 small squares) indicates that the usual delay to conduction between the atria and the ventricles, imposed by the AV junction, has not occurred. This happens if depolarization *originates* in the AV junction, so that it travels up to the atria and down to the ventricles simultaneously, or if it originates as normal in the sinus node but bypasses the AV junction via an *additional faster-conducting pathway*.

A short PR interval should therefore prompt you to think of:

- AV junctional rhythm
- Wolff–Parkinson–White (WPW) syndrome
- Lown–Ganong–levine (LGL) syndrome.

Details of how to recognize and manage each of these are given on the following pages.

Atrioventricular junctional rhythms

If depolarization is initiated from within the AV junction, the wave of atrial depolarization will travel backwards through the atria at the same time as setting off forwards through the AV junction towards the ventricles. Thus, the time delay between atrial depolarization (the P wave) and ventricular depolarization (the QRS complex) will be reduced (Fig. 6.2).

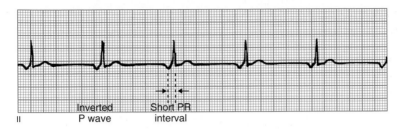

II | Inverted P wave | Short PR interval

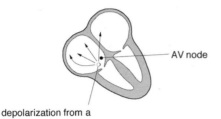

depolarization from a
focus near the AV node

AV node

Fig. 6.2 Depolarization from a
focus near the AV node
Key points:
• P waves inverted in lead II
• PR interval abnormally short

Any source of depolarization within the AV junction can
therefore cause a short PR interval, including:

● AV junctional escape rhythms
● AV junctional ectopics
● AV re-entry tachycardia.

A discussion of how to identify and manage all of these
rhythms can be found in Chapter 3. Atrial ectopics arising near
to the AV node will also have a shorter PR interval than
normal sinus beats, but it will rarely be less than 0.12 s long.

Wolff–Parkinson–White syndrome

In most people, conduction of electricity through the heart
follows just one distinct path from atria to ventricles: namely,
via the AV node, bundle of His and Purkinje fibres. Some
people have an additional connection between the atria and
the ventricles – this is WPW syndrome (Fig. 6.3).

The accessory pathway (called the bundle of Kent) conducts
more quickly than the AV node, so the wave of depolarization
reaches the ventricles more quickly than usual and thus

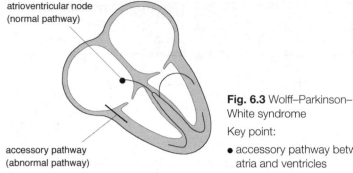

atrioventricular node
(normal pathway)

accessory pathway
(abnormal pathway)

Fig. 6.3 Wolff–Parkinson–
White syndrome
Key point:

• accessory pathway between
atria and ventricles

the PR interval is short. The region of ventricle activated via
the accessory pathway slowly depolarizes, giving rise to a **delta
wave** – the first part of the QRS complex (Fig. 6.4). Shortly
afterwards, the rest of the ventricular muscle is depolarized
rapidly with the arrival of the normally conducted wave of
depolarization via the AV node.

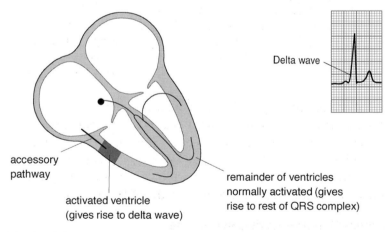

Delta wave

accessory
pathway

activated ventricle
(gives rise to delta wave)

remainder of ventricles
normally activated (gives
rise to rest of QRS complex)

Fig. 6.4 Delta wave
Key point: • the slurred upstroke of the QRS complex is the delta wave

Figure 6.5 shows a 12-lead ECG recorded from a patient with
WPW syndrome.

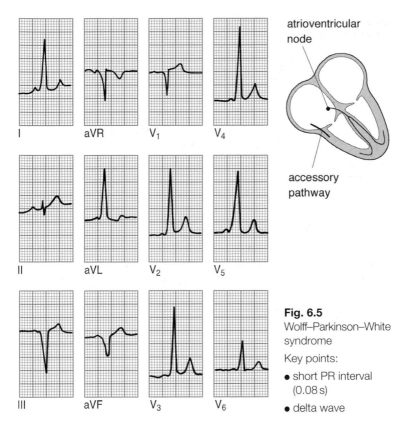

atrioventricular
node

accessory
pathway

Fig. 6.5
Wolff–Parkinson–White
syndrome
Key points:
- short PR interval
  (0.08 s)
- delta wave

WPW syndrome may be found incidentally and be
asymptomatic – if so, no action is needed. Some patients
develop palpitations due to an arrhythmia. The management of
arrhythmias in WPW syndrome is discussed in detail on p. 51.
If a patient with WPW syndrome requires surgery of any kind,
the anaesthetist must be informed of the ECG findings.

Lown–Ganong–Levine syndrome

Patients with LGL syndrome also have an accessory pathway
(called the bundle of James). Unlike the bundle of Kent in
WPW syndrome, however, the bundle of James does not
activate the ventricular muscle directly. Instead, it simply
connects the atria to the bundle of His (Fig. 6.6).

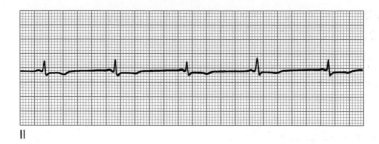

II

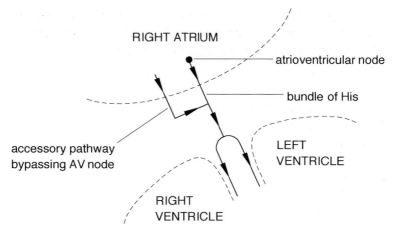

Fig. 6.6 Lown–Ganong–Levine syndrome
Key points: • short PR interval (0.08 s)
                    • no delta wave

Because the accessory bundle allows the wave of depolarization to bypass the slowly conducting AV node, patients with LGL syndrome have a short PR interval. However, as there is no abnormal ventricular activation, there is no delta wave. LGL syndrome carries the same risk of paroxysmal tachycardias as WPW syndrome.

 SEEK HELP

Referral to a cardiologist is appropriate if a patient with a short PR interval has experienced palpitations.

IS THE PR INTERVAL MORE THAN 0.2 SECONDS LONG?

Prolongation of the PR interval is a common finding and indicates that conduction through the AV node has been delayed. When this delay is constant for each cardiac cycle, and each P wave is followed by a QRS complex, it is referred to as **first-degree AV block**.

First-degree AV block is normal when it accompanies a vagally induced bradycardia, as an increase in vagal tone decreases AV nodal conduction. It may also be a feature of:

- ischaemic heart disease
- hypokalaemia
- acute rheumatic myocarditis
- Lyme disease
- drugs
  - digoxin
  - quinidine
  - beta blockers
  - certain calcium-channel blockers.

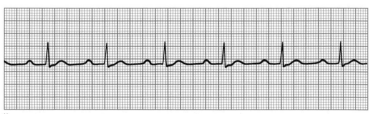

II

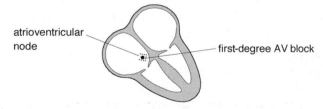

atrioventricular node

first-degree AV block

Fig. 6.7 First-degree AV block

Key point: ● long PR interval (0.31 s)

Figure 6.7 shows a rhythm strip from a patient with first-degree AV block.

Look for a cause by taking a thorough patient history and, in particular, asking about any drug treatment the patient is currently receiving.

First-degree AV block in itself is asymptomatic and, in general, does not progress to other sorts of heart block (described later). No specific treatment is necessary for first-degree AV block *in its own right*, but it should alert you to one of the above diagnoses (which may require treatment). It is *not* an indication for a pacemaker.

DOES THE PR INTERVAL VARY OR CAN IT NOT BE MEASURED?

Normally, the PR interval is constant. In some conditions, however, the interval between P waves and QRS complexes changes, giving rise to a variable PR interval. Sometimes a P wave is not followed by a QRS complex at all and so the PR interval cannot be measured.

If either, or both, of these occur, they indicate one of a number of possible AV conduction problems. These are distinguished by the relationship between P waves and QRS complexes.

- If the PR interval gradually lengthens with each beat, until one P wave fails to produce a QRS complex, the patient has **Mobitz type I AV block**.
- If the PR interval is fixed and normal, but occasionally a P wave fails to produce a QRS complex, the patient has **Mobitz type II AV block**.
- If alternate P waves are not followed by QRS complexes, the patient has **2:1 AV block**.
- If there is no relationship between P waves and QRS complexes, the patient has **third-degree (complete) AV block**.

All three types of AV block are discussed, with example ECGs, on the following pages.

Mobitz type I AV block

Mobitz type I AV block is one of the types of second-degree heart block and is also known as the Wenckebach phenomenon. Its characteristic features are:

● The PR interval shows progressive lengthening until one P wave fails to be conducted and fails to produce a QRS complex.
● The PR interval resets to normal and the cycle repeats.

These features are demonstrated in the rhythm strip in Fig. 6.8.

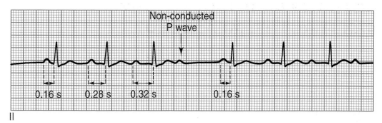

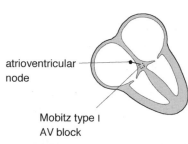

Mobitz type I
AV block

atrioventricular node

Fig. 6.8 Mobitz type I AV block
Key points:
● progressive lengthening of PR interval
● a P wave then fails to be conducted
● PR interval resets and cycle repeats

Mobitz type I AV block is thought to result from abnormal conduction through the AV node itself and can result simply from periods of high vagal activity, so it sometimes occurs during sleep. It may also occur in generalized disease of the conducting tissues. It is regarded as a relatively benign form of AV block, and a permanent pacemaker is not required unless

the frequency of 'dropped' ventricular beats causes a
symptomatic bradycardia.

In acute myocardial infarction, however, pacing may be
required, depending upon the type of infarction. In **anterior**
myocardial infarction, a prophylactic temporary pacemaker is
recommended in case third-degree (complete) heart block
develops. In **inferior** myocardial infarction, a pacemaker
is only needed if symptoms or haemodynamic compromise
result. Patients found to have Mobitz type I AV block
prior to surgery will usually require temporary pacing
perioperatively – discuss this with the anaesthetist and
a cardiologist.

 SEEK HELP

Mobitz type I AV block may require pacing prior to surgery.
Seek the advice of a cardiologist without delay.

Mobitz type II AV block

Mobitz type II AV block is another type of second-degree heart
block and its characteristic features are:

● Most P waves are followed by a QRS complex.
● The PR interval is normal and constant.
● Occasionally, a P wave is not followed by a
  QRS complex.

These features are demonstrated in the rhythm strip in
Fig. 6.9.

Mobitz type II AV block is thought to result from abnormal
conduction below the AV node, in the bundle of His, and is
considered more serious than Mobitz type I as it can progress
without warning to third-degree (complete) heart block.
Referral to a cardiologist is therefore recommended, as a
pacemaker may be required.

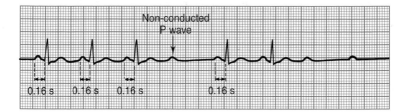

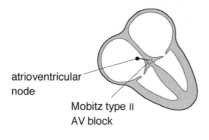

atrioventricular
node

Mobitz type II
AV block

Fig. 6.9 Mobitz type II AV block
Key points:
• PR interval normal and constant
• an occasional P wave fails to be
  conducted

The indications for pacing Mobitz type II AV block in the
setting of an acute MI, or perioperatively, are the same as for
Mobitz type I AV block.

 SEEK HELP

Mobitz type II AV block may require pacing. Seek the advice of
a cardiologist without delay.

2:1 AV block

2:1 AV block is a special form of second-degree heart block
in which alternate P waves are not followed by QRS complexes
(Fig. 6.10).

2:1 AV block cannot be categorized as Mobitz type I or
type II because it is impossible to say whether the
PR interval for the non-conducted P waves would
have been the same as, or longer than, the conducted
P waves.

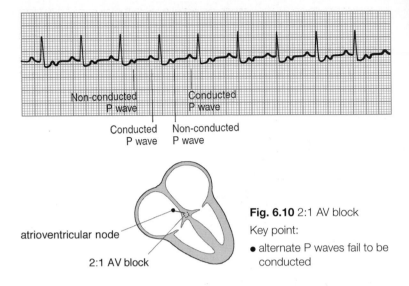

Fig. 6.10 2:1 AV block

Key point:
- alternate P waves fail to be conducted

atrioventricular node

2:1 AV block

Third-degree AV block

In third-degree AV block ('complete heart block'), there is complete interruption of conduction between atria and ventricles, so that the two are working independently. The atrial P waves bear no relationship to the ventricular QRS complexes, which usually arise as the result of a ventricular escape rhythm (p. 58). An example is shown in Fig. 6.11.

It is important to remember that any atrial rhythm can coexist with third-degree heart block, and so the P waves may be abnormal or even absent. A combination of bradycardia (usually 15–40 beats/min) and broad QRS complexes should alert you to suspect third-degree heart block.

In acute **inferior** wall myocardial infarction, third-degree AV block requires pacing if the patient is symptomatic or haemodynamically compromised. In acute **anterior** wall myocardial infarction, the development of third-degree AV block usually indicates an extensive infarct (and thus a poor prognosis). Temporary pacing is indicated regardless of the patient's symptoms or haemodynamic state. Temporary pacing

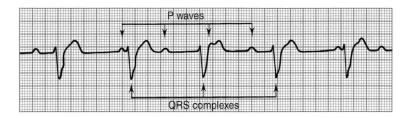

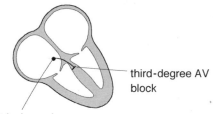

third-degree AV
block

atrioventricular node

Fig. 6.11 Third-degree AV block

Key points:　● P wave (atrial) rate is 85/min

● QRS complex (ventricular) rate is 54/min

● broad QRS complexes

● no relationship between P waves and QRS complexes

is also usually necessary perioperatively in patients about to undergo surgery who are found to have third-degree AV block.

In the elderly, third-degree AV block may cause heart failure, dizziness, falls or even loss of consciousness – permanent pacing is indicated under these circumstances.

Congenital varieties of third-degree AV block are uncommon and you should seek the advice of a cardiologist. In a young patient with a recent onset of third-degree AV block, always consider the possibility of Lyme disease. This is transmitted by the spirochaete *Borrelia burgdorferi* and, in the second stage of the illness, can lead to first-degree, second-degree or third-degree AV block. The AV block can resolve entirely in response to antibiotics, although the patient may require support with a temporary pacemaker during treatment.

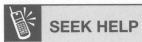

SEEK HELP

Third-degree AV block usually requires pacing. Seek the advice of a cardiologist without delay.

AV dissociation

AV dissociation is a term that is commonly used interchangeably with third-degree AV block; however, it does *not* mean the same thing. AV dissociation should only be used to describe the appearance of an escape rhythm (from the AV junction or ventricles) during sinus bradycardia. This can be distinguished from third-degree AV block by recognizing that the ventricular (QRS) rate is *higher* than the atrial (P wave) rate. The opposite is found in third-degree AV block.

Summary

To assess the PR interval, ask the following questions:

1. Is the PR interval less than 0.12 s long?

If 'yes', consider:
- AV junctional rhythms
- WPW syndrome
- LGL syndrome.

2. Is the PR interval more than 0.2 s long?

If 'yes', consider:
- first-degree AV block
  - ischaemic heart disease
  - hypokalaemia
  - acute rheumatic myocarditis
  - Lyme disease
  - drugs
    digoxin
    quinidine
    beta blockers
    certain calcium-channel blockers.

3. Does the PR interval vary or can it not be measured?

If 'yes', consider:
- second-degree AV block
  - Mobitz type I (Wenckebach phenomenon)
  - Mobitz type II
  - 2:1 AV block
- third-degree AV block.

7

THE Q WAVE

After measuring the PR interval, go on to examine the QRS complex in each lead. Begin by looking for Q waves. A Q wave is present whenever the first deflection of the QRS complex points downwards (Fig. 7.1).

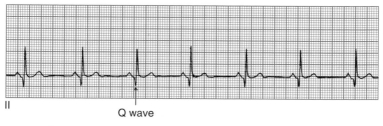

II

Q wave

Fig. 7.1 The Q wave

Key point: ● Q wave is present when the first QRS deflection is downwards

As you examine the QRS complex in each lead, the first question to ask is:

● Are there any 'pathological' Q waves?

In this chapter we will help you to answer this question and to interpret any abnormality you may find.

ARE THERE ANY 'PATHOLOGICAL' Q WAVES?

If Q waves are present, begin by asking:

● Could these be normal?

Q waves are usually absent from *most* of the leads of a normal ECG. However, *small* Q waves are normal in leads that look at the heart from the left: I, II, aVL, V_5 and V_6. They result from septal depolarization, which normally occurs from left to right, and hence are referred to as 'septal' Q waves (Fig. 7.2).

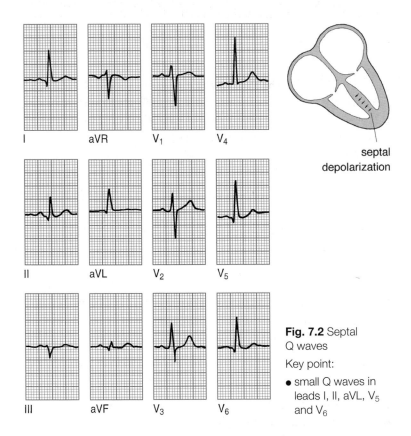

septal
depolarization

Fig. 7.2 Septal Q waves

Key point:

- small Q waves in leads I, II, aVL, V_5 and V_6

A small Q wave may also be normal in lead III, and is often associated with an inverted T wave. Both may disappear on deep inspiration (Fig. 7.3).

Q waves in other leads are likely to be abnormal or **'pathological'**, particularly if they are:

- >2 small squares deep, or

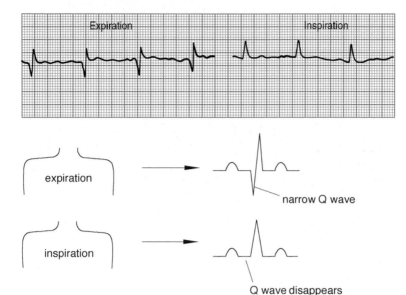

Fig. 7.3 Normal Q waves in lead III

Key points: ● narrow Q waves in lead III

● disappear on inspiration

● >25 per cent of the height of the following R wave in depth, and/or
● >1 small square wide.

If wide or deep Q waves (i.e. exceeding the above criteria) are present, consider:

● myocardial infarction
● left ventricular hypertrophy
● bundle branch block.

Myocardial infarction and left ventricular hypertrophy are discussed on the following pages. The bundle branch blocks are covered in detail in Chapter 8.

An abnormal Q wave (in lead III) is also a feature of:

● pulmonary embolism.

It is part of the 'classic' $S_IQ_{III}T_{III}$ pattern that is often quoted, although rarely seen. However, the Q_{III} rarely satisfies the 'pathological' Q wave criteria. The most frequent finding in pulmonary embolism is a tachycardia.

Myocardial infarction

Q waves start to appear within a few hours of the onset of myocardial infarction and in 90 per cent of cases become permanent. The presence of Q waves alone therefore gives no clue as to the timing of the infarction. As with the other ECG changes in myocardial infarction, the location of the infarction can be determined from an analysis of the ECG leads (see Table 9.2).

Figure 7.4 shows an ECG recorded 5 days after an anterior myocardial infarction. Q waves have developed in leads V_1–V_4.

Figure 7.5 is from a patient who had an inferior myocardial infarction 2 years previously. Abnormal Q waves are seen in leads II, III and aVF.

The diagnosis of acute myocardial infarction is normally apparent from the presenting symptoms (chest pain, nausea and sweating) and ECG changes that are present (especially ST segment elevation), and can be confirmed by serial cardiac enzyme measurements. The management of acute myocardial infarction is discussed in detail in Chapter 9.

 ACT QUICKLY

Acute myocardial infarction is a medical emergency. Prompt diagnosis and treatment are essential.

When Q waves are found 'incidentally' on an ECG recorded for other reasons, a thorough review of the patient's history is

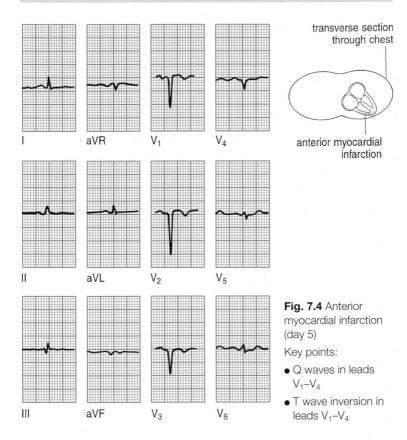

I aVR V₁ V₄

transverse section
through chest

anterior myocardial
infarction

II aVL V₂ V₅

III aVF V₃ V₆

Fig. 7.4 Anterior
myocardial infarction
(day 5)

Key points:

● Q waves in leads
V_1–V_4

● T wave inversion in
leads V_1–V_4

necessary. Ask about:

● previous documented myocardial infarctions
● previous symptoms suggestive of myocardial infarction
● symptoms of recent myocardial ischaemia.

However, bear in mind that approximately 20 per cent of myocardial infarctions are painless or 'silent'. If you remain uncertain about the significance of abnormal Q waves, and are suspicious about a previous myocardial infarction, there are a number of investigations that can help:

● exercise ECG (Chapter 16)
● exercise thallium scintigraphy
● coronary angiography.

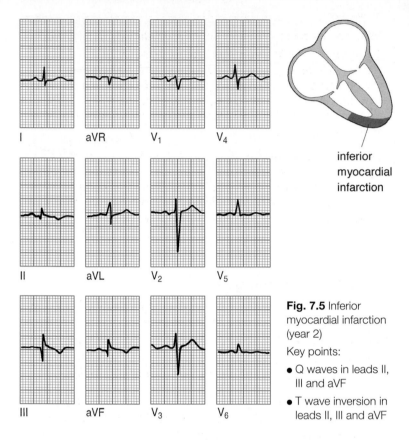

inferior
myocardial
infarction

Fig. 7.5 Inferior
myocardial infarction
(year 2)

Key points:

- Q waves in leads II,
  III and aVF
- T wave inversion in
  leads II, III and aVF

A cardiologist will be able to advise you on which of these
tests, if any, are appropriate.

Why do Q waves appear in myocardial infarction?

Q waves develop in myocardial infarction following the necrosis (death) of an area of myocardium. The leads over the necrosed region can no longer record electrical activity in that area, and so they look 'through' it to record ventricular depolarization from 'within' the ventricular cavity rather than from outside.

Because each wave of depolarization flows from the inner surface of the heart to the outer, a lead recording the depolarization from a viewpoint 'within' the ventricle would 'see' the electrical activity flowing away from it; hence, the negative deflection on the ECG – the Q wave.

Left ventricular hypertrophy

At the start of this chapter, we said that small ('septal') Q waves can be a normal finding and result from depolarization of the interventricular septum. If the septum hypertrophies, its muscle mass (and hence the amount of electricity generated by depolarization) increases, and the Q waves become deeper.

Left ventricular hypertrophy often involves the septum, and so deep Q waves are often seen in leads looking at the left and inferior surfaces of the heart (Fig. 7.6).

Left ventricular hypertrophy is discussed more fully on p. 135.

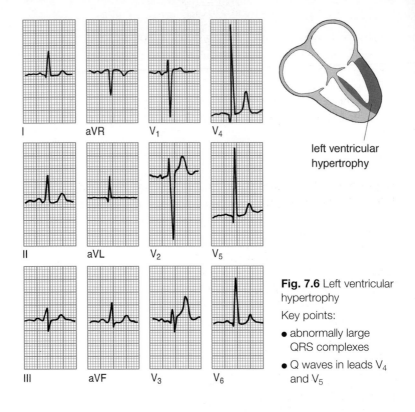

left ventricular
hypertrophy

Fig. 7.6 Left ventricular
hypertrophy

Key points:

- abnormally large
  QRS complexes
- Q waves in leads V_4
  and V_5

Summary

To assess the Q wave, ask the following question:

1. Are there any 'pathological' Q waves?

If 'yes', consider:
- myocardial infarction
- left ventricular hypertrophy
- bundle branch block.

Also:
- pulmonary embolism (although rarely 'pathological').

8

THE QRS COMPLEX

Normal QRS complexes have a different appearance in each of the 12 ECG leads (Fig. 8.1).

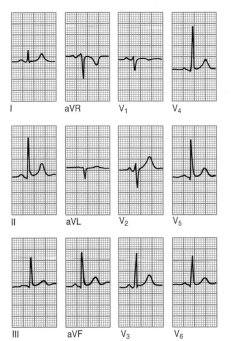

Fig. 8.1 Normal 12-lead ECG
Key point:

● appearance of QRS complex varies from lead to lead

When reviewing an ECG, look carefully at the size and shape of the QRS complexes in each lead and ask yourself the following four questions:

● Are any R or S waves too big?
● Are the QRS complexes too small?

● Are any QRS complexes too wide?
● Are any QRS complexes an abnormal shape?

In this chapter, we will help you to answer these questions and to interpret any abnormalities you may find.

ARE ANY R OR S WAVES TOO BIG?

The height of the R wave and depth of the S wave vary from lead to lead in the normal ECG (as Fig. 8.1 shows). As a rule, in the normal ECG:

● The R wave *increases* in height from lead V_1 to V_6.
● The R wave is *smaller* than the S wave in leads V_1 and V_2.
● The R wave is *bigger* than the S wave in leads V_5 and V_6.
● The tallest R wave does not exceed 25 mm in height.
● The deepest S wave does not exceed 25 mm in depth.

Always look carefully at the R and S waves in each lead, and check whether they conform to these criteria. If not, first of all consider:

● incorrect ECG calibration (should be 1 mV = 10 mm).

If the calibration is correct, consider whether your patient has one of the following:

● left ventricular hypertrophy (LVH)
● right ventricular hypertrophy (RVH)
● posterior myocardial infarction
● Wolff–Parkinson–White (WPW) syndrome
● dextrocardia.

Each of these conditions is discussed on the following pages.

If the QRS complex is also abnormally wide, think of:

● bundle branch block

which is discussed later in this chapter.

Left ventricular hypertrophy

Hypertrophy of the left ventricle causes tall R waves in the leads that 'look at' the left ventricle – namely, I, aVL, V_5 and V_6 – and the reciprocal ('mirror image') change of deep S waves in leads that 'look at' the right ventricle – V_1 and V_2.

LVH should be suspected if *any* of the following criteria are met:

- The R wave in V_5 or V_6 exceeds 25 mm.
- The S wave in V_1 or V_2 exceeds 25 mm.
- The total of the R wave in V_5 or V_6 plus the S wave in V_1 or V_2 exceeds 35 mm.

These criteria are not diagnostic of LVH, as young, thin people with normal hearts often have R and S waves outside these limits.

Figure 8.2 shows the ECG of a patient with LVH.

If evidence of LVH is present on the ECG, look too for evidence of 'strain':

- ST segment depression
- T wave inversion.

See Fig. 9.15 for an example of LVH with 'strain'.

Echocardiography is diagnostic for LVH. The treatment is usually that of the cause (Table 8.1).

Right ventricular hypertrophy

Right ventricular hypertrophy causes a 'dominant' R wave (i.e. bigger than the S wave) in the leads that 'look at' the right ventricle, particularly V_1. RVH is also associated with:

- right axis deviation (Chapter 4)
- deep S waves in leads V_5 and V_6
- right bundle branch block (RBBB)

and, if 'strain' is present:

- ST segment depression
- T wave inversion.

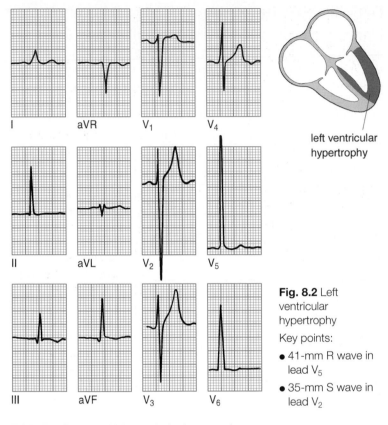

I aVR V_1 V_4

left ventricular hypertrophy

II aVL V_2 V_5

III aVF V_3 V_6

Fig. 8.2 Left ventricular hypertrophy

Key points:
- 41-mm R wave in lead V_5
- 35-mm S wave in lead V_2

Table 8.1 Causes of left ventricular hypertrophy

- Hypertension
- Aortic stenosis
- Coarctation of the aorta
- Hypertrophic cardiomyopathy

Figure 8.3 shows the ECG of a patient with RVH and 'strain'.

If you suspect RVH, look for an underlying cause (Table 8.2). The treatment of RVH is that of the underlying cause.

Posterior myocardial infarction

Posterior myocardial infarction is one of a small number of causes of a 'dominant' R wave in lead V_1 (Table 8.3).

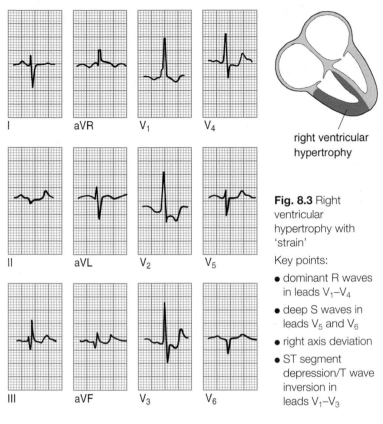

right ventricular hypertrophy

Fig. 8.3 Right ventricular hypertrophy with 'strain'

Key points:

- dominant R waves in leads V_1–V_4
- deep S waves in leads V_5 and V_6
- right axis deviation
- ST segment depression/T wave inversion in leads V_1–V_3

Table 8.2 Causes of right ventricular hypertrophy

- Pulmonary hypertension
- Pulmonary stenosis

Table 8.3 Causes of a 'dominant' R wave in lead V_1

- Right ventricular hypertrophy
- Posterior myocardial infarction
- Wolff–Parkinson–White syndrome (left-sided accessory pathway)

Infarction of the posterior wall of the left ventricle leads to reciprocal changes when viewed from the perspective of the anterior chest leads. Thus, the usual appearances of pathological Q waves, ST segment elevation and inverted T waves will appear as *R waves*, ST segment *depression* and *upright, tall* T waves when viewed from leads V_1–V_3 (Fig. 8.4).

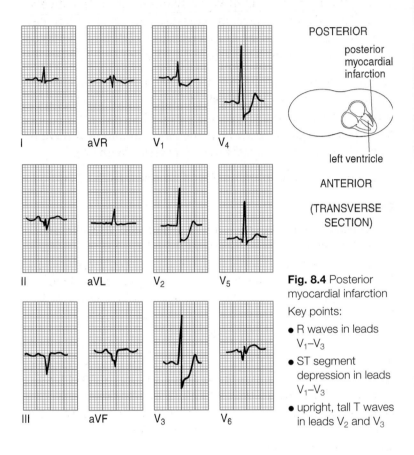

Fig. 8.4 Posterior myocardial infarction

Key points:
- R waves in leads V_1–V_3
- ST segment depression in leads V_1–V_3
- upright, tall T waves in leads V_2 and V_3

The management of acute myocardial infarction is discussed in detail in Chapter 9.

 ACT QUICKLY

Acute myocardial infarction is a medical emergency. Prompt diagnosis and treatment are essential.

Wolf–Parkinson–White syndrome

If you see a dominant R wave in leads V_1-V_3 in the presence of a short PR interval, think of WPW syndrome (p. 111). Patients with WPW syndrome have an accessory pathway (the bundle of Kent) that bypasses the atrioventricular node and bundle of His to connect the atria directly to the ventricles.

Accurate localization of the position of the accessory pathway can only be made with electrophysiological studies. Generally, however, a dominant R wave in leads V_1-V_3 indicates a left-sided accessory pathway, whereas a dominant S wave in leads V_1-V_3 indicates a right-sided accessory pathway.

The management of WPW syndrome is discussed in Chapter 6.

Dextrocardia

In dextrocardia, the heart lies on the right side of the chest instead of the left. The ECG does not show the normal progressive increase in R wave height across the chest leads; instead, the QRS complexes decrease in height across them (Fig. 8.5). In addition, the P wave is inverted in lead I and there is right axis deviation. **Right-sided chest leads** will show the pattern normally seen on the left.

If you suspect dextrocardia, check the location of the patient's apex beat. A chest X-ray is diagnostic. No specific treatment is required for dextrocardia, but ensure the condition is highlighted in the patient's notes and check for any associated syndromes (e.g. Kartagener's syndrome – dextrocardia, bronchiectasis and sinusitis).

ARE THE QRS COMPLEXES TOO SMALL?

Small QRS complexes indicate that relatively little of the voltage generated by ventricular depolarization is reaching the ECG electrodes. Although criteria exist for the normal upper limit of QRS complex size, there are no similar guidelines for the lower limit of QRS size.

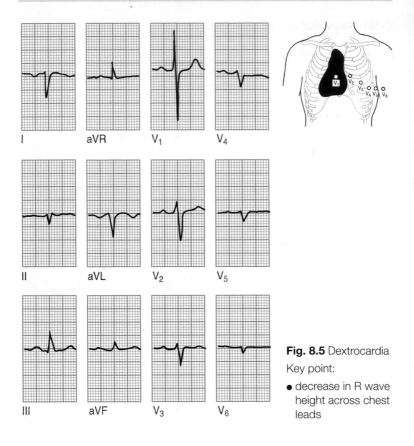

Fig. 8.5 Dextrocardia

Key point:

- decrease in R wave height across chest leads

Small QRS complexes may simply reflect a variant of normal. However, always check for:

- incorrect ECG calibration (should be 1 mV = 10 mm)

and also check whether the patient has:

- obesity
- emphysema.

Both of these conditions increase the distance between the heart and the chest electrodes.

However, if the QRS complexes appear small, and particularly if they have changed in relation to earlier ECG recordings, always consider the possibility of:

● pericardial effusion.

This is discussed on the following pages.

Pericardial effusion

A pericardial effusion reduces the voltage of the QRS complexes (Fig. 8.6).

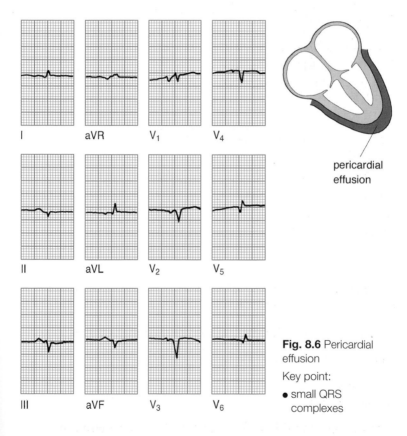

Fig. 8.6 Pericardial effusion

Key point:

● small QRS complexes

Pericardial effusion can also cause electrical alternans, in which the height of the R waves and/or T waves alternates from beat to beat (Fig. 8.7).

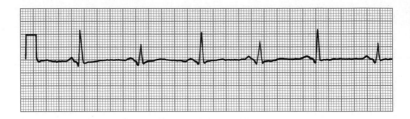

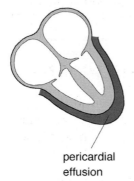

pericardial
effusion

Fig. 8.7 Electrical alternans in pericardial effusion

Key point:

● variation in beat-to-beat R wave height

A pericardial effusion may be asymptomatic when small. Larger effusions cause breathlessness and, ultimately, cardiac tamponade. The signs of Beck's triad indicate significant cardiac compromise:

● low blood pressure
● elevated jugular venous pressure
● impalpable apex beat.

In addition, the heart sounds are soft and there may be pulsus paradoxus (a marked fall in blood pressure on inspiration). The combination of small QRS complexes, electrical alternans and a tachycardia is a highly specific, but insensitive, indicator of a pericardial tamponade.

In a patient with a pericardial effusion, the chest X-ray may show a large globular heart but with no distension of the pulmonary veins. The echocardiogram is diagnostic.

Obtain the advice of a cardiologist immediately, particularly if the effusion is causing haemodynamic impairment. Urgent pericardial aspiration is required if the signs of tamponade are present, but should only be undertaken by, or under the guidance of, someone experienced in the procedure.

 ACT QUICKLY

Cardiac tamponade is a medical emergency. Prompt diagnosis and treatment are essential.

ARE ANY QRS COMPLEXES TOO WIDE?

The QRS complex corresponds to depolarization of the ventricles, and this normally takes no longer than 0.12 s from start to finish. Thus, the width of a normal QRS complex is no greater than 3 small squares on the ECG.

Widening of the QRS complex is seen if conduction through the ventricles is slower than normal, and this usually means that depolarization has taken an abnormal route through the ventricles, as happens in:

- bundle branch block
- ventricular rhythms.

These conditions are discussed on the following pages.

Widening of the QRS complex can also result from the abnormal mechanism of depolarization that occurs with:

- hyperkalaemia.

Hyperkalaemia is discussed in detail on p. 178.

Bundle branch block

After leaving the bundle of His, the conduction fibres divide into two separate pathways as they pass through the interventricular septum – the left and right bundle branches – which supply the left and right ventricles respectively.

A block of either of the bundle branches delays the electrical activation of its ventricle, which must instead be depolarized *indirectly* via the other bundle branch. This prolongs the process of ventricular depolarization, and so the QRS complex is wider than 3 small squares. In addition, the shape of the QRS complex is distorted because of the abnormal pathway of depolarization.

In **left bundle branch block** (LBBB), the interventricular septum has to depolarize from right to left, a reversal of the normal pattern. This causes a small Q wave in lead V_1 and a small R wave in lead V_6 (Fig. 8.8). The right ventricle is depolarized normally via the right bundle branch, causing an R wave in lead V_1 and an S wave in lead V_6 (Fig. 8.9). Then, the left ventricle is depolarized by the right, causing an S wave in lead V_1 and another R wave (called R') in lead V_6 (Fig. 8.10).

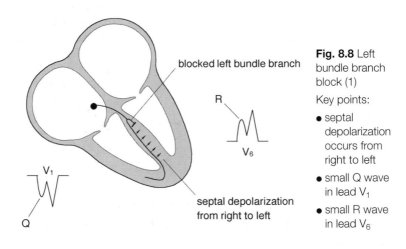

blocked left bundle branch

R

V_6

V_1

Q

septal depolarization from right to left

Fig. 8.8 Left bundle branch block (1)

Key points:

- septal depolarization occurs from right to left

- small Q wave in lead V_1

- small R wave in lead V_6

Thus, the ECG of a patient with LBBB appears as in Fig. 8.11.

In **right bundle branch block,** the interventricular septum depolarizes normally, from left to right, causing a tiny R wave in lead V_1 and a small 'septal' Q wave in lead V_6 (Fig. 8.12).

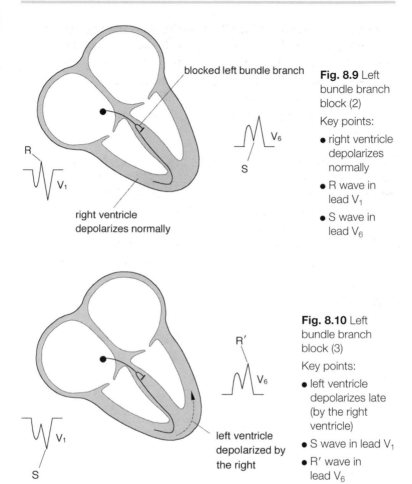

Fig. 8.9 Left bundle branch block (2)

Key points:

- right ventricle depolarizes normally
- R wave in lead V_1
- S wave in lead V_6

Fig. 8.10 Left bundle branch block (3)

Key points:

- left ventricle depolarizes late (by the right ventricle)
- S wave in lead V_1
- R′ wave in lead V_6

The left ventricle is depolarized normally via the left bundle branch, causing an S wave in lead V_1 and an R wave in lead V_6 (Fig. 8.13).

Then, the right ventricle is depolarized by the left, causing another R wave (called R′) in lead V_1 and an S wave in lead V_6 (Fig. 8.14).

Thus, the ECG of a patient with RBBB appears as in Fig. 8.15.

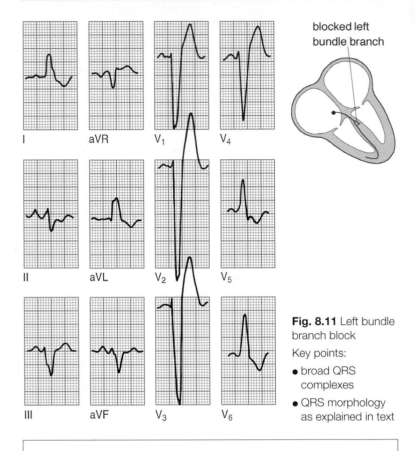

Fig. 8.11 Left bundle branch block

Key points:
- broad QRS complexes
- QRS morphology as explained in text

An aide-memoire

Remembering the name 'William Morrow' should help you recall that:
- In LBBB, the QRS looks like a 'W' in lead V_1 and an 'M' in lead V_6 (**Willia**m).
- In RBBB, the QRS looks like an 'M' in lead V_1 and a 'W' in lead V_6 (**Morro**w).

The presence of LBBB is almost invariably an indication of underlying pathology (Table 8.4), and the patient should be assessed accordingly. LBBB can be the presenting ECG feature of acute myocardial infarction, and is an indication for

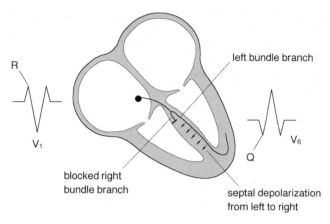

Fig. 8.12 Right bundle branch block (1)

Key points: • septum depolarization occurs from left to right

• small R wave in lead V_1

• small 'septal' Q wave in lead V_6

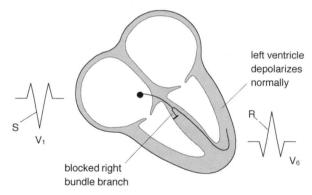

Fig. 8.13 Right bundle branch block (2)

Key points: • left ventricle depolarizes normally

• S wave in lead V_1

• R wave in lead V_6

thrombolysis. The presence of LBBB renders interpretation of the ECG beyond the QRS complex impossible.

In contrast to LBBB, RBBB is a relatively common finding in otherwise normal hearts. However, it too can result from

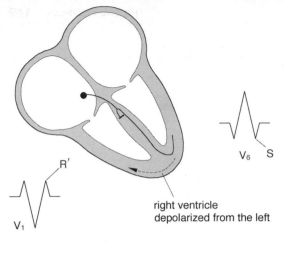

Fig. 8.14 Right bundle branch block (3)

Key points:
- right ventricle depolarizes late (by the left ventricle)
- R' wave in lead V_1
- S wave in lead V_6

right ventricle depolarized from the left

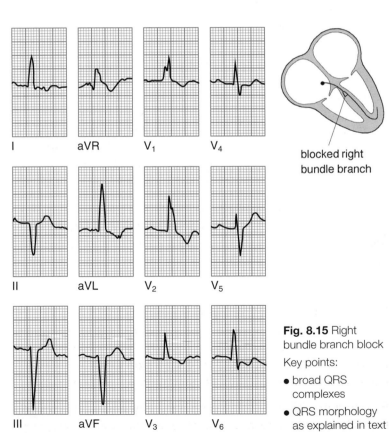

blocked right bundle branch

Fig. 8.15 Right bundle branch block

Key points:
- broad QRS complexes
- QRS morphology as explained in text

Table 8.4 Causes of left bundle branch block

- Ischaemic heart disease
- Cardiomyopathy
- Left ventricular hypertrophy
  - hypertension
  - aortic stenosis
- Fibrosis of the conduction system

underlying disease (Table 8.5) and should be investigated according to the clinical presentation.

Table 8.5 Causes of right bundle branch block

- Ischaemic heart disease
- Cardiomyopathy
- Atrial septal defect
- Ebstein's anomaly
- Pulmonary embolism (usually massive)

Bundle branch block (particularly RBBB) can also occur at fast heart rates. This is not uncommonly seen during supraventricular tachycardia (SVT), and the resultant broad complexes can lead to an incorrect diagnosis of ventricular tachycardia (VT) by the unwary. For help in distinguishing between VT and SVT, turn to p. 73.

Both LBBB and RBBB are asymptomatic in themselves, and do not require treatment in their own right. Even so, they should prompt you to look for an underlying cause that is appropriate to the patient's presentation.

Ventricular rhythms

When depolarization is initiated from within the ventricular muscle itself, the wave of electrical activity has to spread from myocyte to myocyte rather than using the more rapid Purkinje network. This prolongs the process of ventricular depolarization and thus widens the QRS complex (Fig. 8.16).

For more information about ventricular rhythms, and help with their identification, turn to Chapter 3.

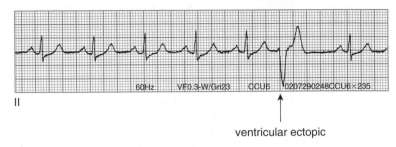

ventricular ectopic

Fig. 8.16 Ventricular ectopic

Key points: ● broad QRS complex

● complex occurs earlier than expected

ARE ANY QRS COMPLEXES AN ABNORMAL SHAPE?

Most of the causes of an abnormally shaped QRS complex have been discussed earlier in this chapter. However, occasionally you will encounter QRS complexes that just appear unusual without fitting any of these specific criteria.

You may see complexes which appear 'slurred', or have an abnormal 'notch', without necessarily being abnormally tall, small or wide. If this is the case, consider the following possible causes:

● incomplete bundle branch block
● fascicular block
● WPW syndrome.

Further information on each of these can be found on the following pages.

Incomplete bundle branch block

Bundle branch block is discussed earlier in this chapter. Sometimes, however, conduction down a bundle branch can be *delayed* without being blocked entirely. When this happens, the QRS complex develops an abnormal shape but the complex remains less than 3 small squares wide. This is called

incomplete (or partial) bundle branch block, and can affect
either left or right bundle branches (Figs 8.17 and 8.18).

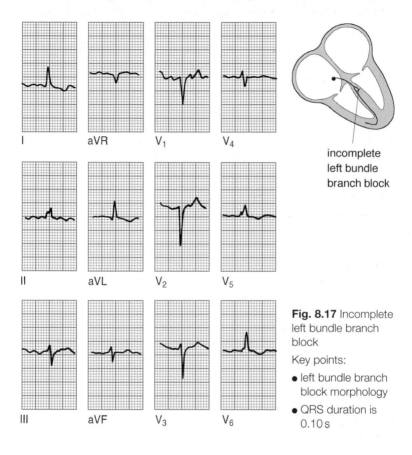

I aVR V$_1$ V$_4$

II aVL V$_2$ V$_5$

III aVF V$_3$ V$_6$

incomplete
left bundle
branch block

Fig. 8.17 Incomplete
left bundle branch
block
Key points:
- left bundle branch
  block morphology
- QRS duration is
  0.10 s

The causes of incomplete bundle branch block are the same as
those of complete bundle branch block, which is discussed
earlier in this chapter.

Fascicular block

Block of one of the two fascicles of the left bundle causes
either left or right axis deviation (Chapter 4). The consequent
delay to conduction may also lead to slurring or notching of
the QRS complex.

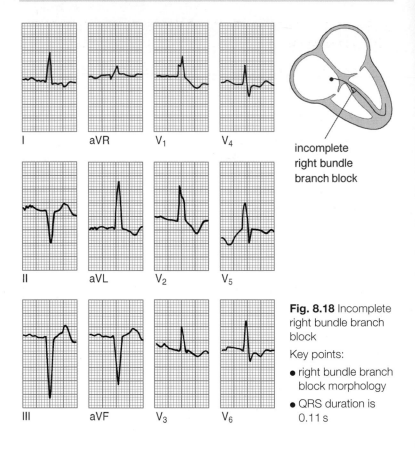

I   aVR V_1 V_4

incomplete right bundle branch block

II   aVL V_2 V_5

Fig. 8.18 Incomplete right bundle branch block

Key points:
- right bundle branch block morphology
- QRS duration is 0.11 s

III   aVF V_3 V_6

How to identify which fascicle is affected, and manage the patient subsequently, is discussed in Chapter 4.

Wolff–Parkinson–White syndrome

Patients with WPW syndrome characteristically exhibit a delta wave that slurs the upstroke of the QRS complex (see Fig. 6.4). This diagnosis should be suspected if, in addition, the PR interval is abnormally short. For more information on the diagnosis and management of WPW syndrome, turn to p. 111.

Summary

To assess the QRS complex, ask the following questions:

1. Are any R or S waves too big?

If 'yes', consider:
- incorrect ECG calibration
- left ventricular hypertrophy
- right ventricular hypertrophy
- posterior myocardial infarction
- WPW syndrome (left-sided accessory pathway)
- dextrocardia.

Also:
- bundle branch block.

2. Are the QRS complexes too small?

If 'yes', consider:
- incorrect ECG calibration
- obesity
- emphysema
- pericardial effusion.

3. Are any QRS complexes too wide?

If 'yes', consider:
- bundle branch block
- ventricular rhythms.

Also:
- hyperkalaemia.

4. Are any QRS complexes an abnormal shape?

If 'yes', consider:
- incomplete bundle branch block
- fascicular block
- WPW syndrome.

9

THE ST SEGMENT

The ST segment lies between the end of the S wave and the start of the T wave. Normally, the ST segment is isoelectric, meaning that it lies at the same level as the ECG's baseline, the horizontal line between the end of the T wave and the start of the P wave (Fig. 9.1).

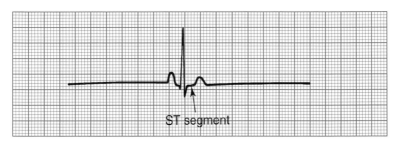

Fig. 9.1 The ST segment

Key point:　● ST segment is normally isoelectric

ST segments can be abnormal in one of two ways, so the questions you need to ask about the ST segments when you review them are:

● Are the ST segments elevated?
● Are the ST segments depressed?

In this chapter, we will help you to answer these questions, and guide you on what to do next if you find an abnormality.

ARE THE ST SEGMENTS ELEVATED?

Look carefully at the ST segment in each lead to see if it is isoelectric. If it is raised above this level, the ST segment is elevated.

ST segment elevation should never be ignored, as it frequently indicates a serious problem that warrants urgent attention. If you see ST elevation in any lead, consider the following possible diagnoses:

- acute myocardial infarction
- left ventricular aneurysm
- Prinzmetal's (vasospastic) angina
- pericarditis
- high take-off.

Therefore, ST segment elevation can represent anything from a potentially life-threatening condition to a normal variant, making it particularly important to identify the cause. To help you in this task, we describe each of these five conditions (together with example ECGs) on the pages that follow.

Acute myocardial infarction

By definition, myocardial infarction causes permanent damage to the heart muscle. Myocardial infarction may be classified into:

- Q wave infarcts or ST segment elevation myocardial infarction (STEMI)
- non-Q wave infarcts or non-ST segment elevation myocardial infarction (NSTEMI).

This section is chiefly concerned with Q wave infarction (STEMI). Further information about non-Q wave infarction (NSTEMI) can be found in Chapter 10.

In Q wave myocardial infarction (STEMI), the ECG changes gradually 'evolve' in the sequence shown in Fig. 9.2. The earliest change is ST segment elevation accompanied, or even preceded, by tall 'hyperacute' T waves. Over the next few hours or days, Q waves appear, the ST segments return to normal and the T waves become inverted. It is usual for some permanent abnormality of the ECG to persist following myocardial infarction – usually 'pathological' Q waves, although the T waves may remain inverted permanently too.

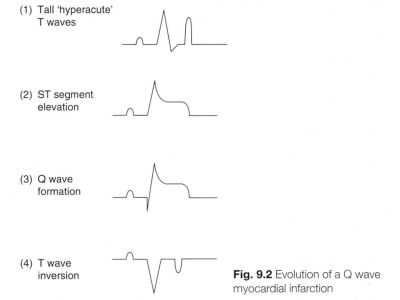

(1) Tall 'hyperacute' T waves

(2) ST segment elevation

(3) Q wave formation

(4) T wave inversion

Fig. 9.2 Evolution of a Q wave myocardial infarction

Do not forget that acute myocardial infarction can also present with the new onset of left bundle branch block on the ECG (Chapter 8). Remember too that a normal ECG does not exclude an acute myocardial infarction.

Acute myocardial infarction requires urgent treatment and you must lose no time in trying to make the diagnosis. The diagnosis is established if at least two of the following three criteria are consistent with a myocardial infarction:

● patient's history
● ECG changes
● changes in cardiac markers.

The symptoms of myocardial infarction are:

- tight, central chest pain
- nausea and vomiting
- sweating.

The pain is more severe, and longer lasting, than that of angina. Always ask about a history of previous angina or myocardial infarction and assess cardiac risk factors (Table 9.1) and any possible contraindications to aspirin or thrombolysis. A thorough clinical examination is mandatory.

Table 9.1 Risk factors for coronary artery disease

Modifiable:
- Cigarette smoking
- Hypertension
- Diabetes mellitus
- Hyperlipidaemia

Non-modifiable:
- Age
- Male sex
- Family history

Aortic dissection

Always beware of missing a diagnosis of aortic dissection. This too can cause ST segment elevation (if the dissection involves the coronary arteries) and chest pain, but patients may also complain of a 'tearing' back pain, have a different blood pressure in each arm and have mediastinal widening on their chest X-ray.

Cardiac markers commonly measured in myocardial infarction are:

- troponins I and T
- creatine kinase (CK) or its isoenzyme CK-MB (which is more cardiac specific)
- aspartate transaminase (AST) and lactate dehydrogenase (LDH).

Troponins are relatively sensitive and specific markers of myocyte necrosis. The isoenzyme CK-MB is more cardiac specific than CK, AST or LDH.

Cardiac markers peak at different times after the onset of the infarction (Fig. 9.3). You can see from Fig. 9.3 that significant changes in the cardiac enzymes may not be apparent for several hours after the onset of an infarction. Cardiac markers therefore have little role to play in the initial diagnosis of a myocardial infarction, and it is not at all unusual for levels to be normal upon admission.

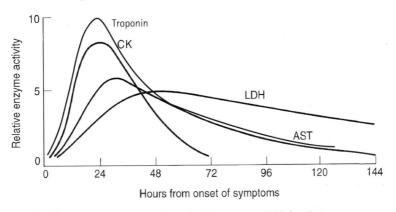

Fig. 9.3 Time course of enzyme levels after myocardial infarction

Key points:
- Troponins peak after 12 h
- CK peaks after 24 h
- AST peaks after 30 h
- LDH peaks after 48 h

Having diagnosed myocardial infarction, waste no time in admitting the patient to a coronary care unit or other monitored area for treatment as indicated. This is discussed later in this section.

The ECG also allows you to identify the area of myocardium damaged by the infarction, as the leads 'looking at' that area will be the ones in which abnormalities are seen (Table 9.2). Examples of myocardial infarctions affecting different areas are shown in Figs 9.4–9.6.

Table 9.2 Localization of myocardial infarctions

Leads containing ST segment elevation	Location of myocardial infarction
V_1–V_4	Anterior myocardial infarction
I, aVL, V_5–V_6	Lateral myocardial infarction
I, aVL, V_1–V_6	Anterolateral myocardial infarction
V_1–V_3	Anteroseptal myocardial infarction
II, III, aVF	Inferior myocardial infarction
I, aVL, V_5–V_6, II, III, aVF	Inferolateral myocardial infarction

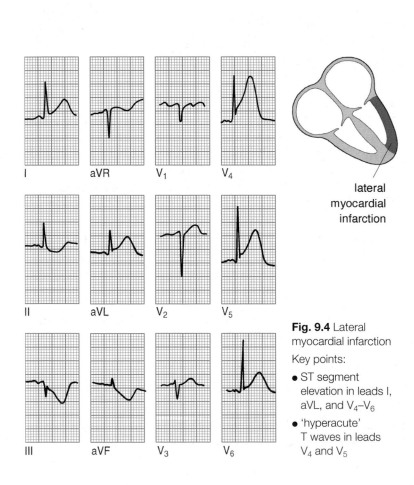

lateral
myocardial
infarction

Fig. 9.4 Lateral
myocardial infarction
Key points:

- ST segment
  elevation in leads I,
  aVL, and V_4–V_6
- 'hyperacute'
  T waves in leads
  V_4 and V_5

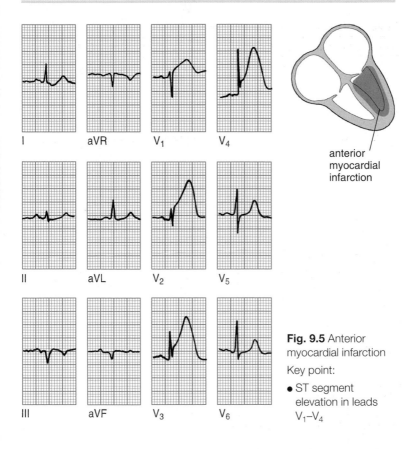

I aVR V₁ V₄

anterior
myocardial
infarction

II aVL V₂ V₅

III aVF V₃ V₆

Fig. 9.5 Anterior
myocardial infarction

Key point:

● ST segment
elevation in leads
V₁–V₄

If you diagnose an inferior myocardial infarction, you must go
on to ask the question:

● Is the right ventricle involved?

To make the diagnosis, you must perform another ECG, but this
time use right-sided chest leads (Fig. 9.7). Look for ST segment
elevation in lead V₄R (Fig. 9.8). If present, there is a high
likelihood of right ventricular involvement.

Why is right ventricular infarction important?

Patients with a right ventricular infarction may develop the signs of right-sided heart failure (elevated jugular venous pressure and peripheral oedema). The left ventricle may be functioning normally, so the lungs are clear. If these patients develop hypotension, it is usually because their left-sided filling pressure is too low (as the supply of blood from the damaged right ventricle is inadequate). Vasodilator drugs must be avoided. Intravenous fluids may be needed to maintain right ventricular output, thus ensuring sufficient blood is supplied to the left ventricle.

It may seem paradoxical to give intravenous fluids to patients who already appear to be in right heart failure, unless the reasons for doing so are understood. If haemodynamically compromised, these patients need fluid balance monitoring using a Swan–Ganz catheter, which measures right-sided and, indirectly, left-sided filling pressure. The risk of severe complications is high in these patients.

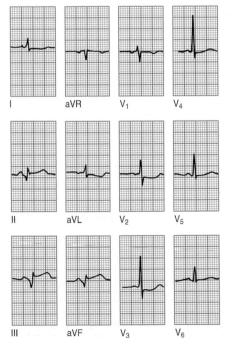

Fig. 9.6 Inferior myocardial infarction

Key points:

- Q waves in leads II, III and aVF
- ST segment elevation in leads II, III and aVF

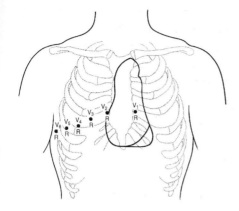

Fig. 9.7 Positioning of right-sided chest leads

Patients with acute myocardial infarction require:

- pain relief (an opiate intravenously and an anti-emetic)
- oxygen
- aspirin, 300 mg orally.

Unless contraindicated, thrombolysis should be offered to all patients whose history suggests a myocardial infarction within the last 12 h and whose ECG shows:

- ST segment elevation consistent with infarction, or
- new left bundle branch block.

Following a myocardial infarction, patients should continue with:

- aspirin, 75 mg daily
- a beta blocker (e.g. timolol, 5 mg twice daily)
- an angiotensin-converting enzyme inhibitor if evidence of heart failure appears during the hospital stay
- a statin.

 ACT QUICKLY

Acute myocardial infarction is a medical emergency. Prompt diagnosis and treatment are essential.

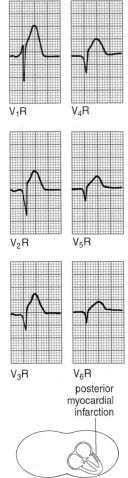

V₁R   V₄R

V₂R   V₅R

V₃R   V₆R
       posterior
       myocardial
       infarction

Fig. 9.8 Right ventricular involvement

Key points:

- only right-sided chest leads are shown
- ST segment elevation in all leads (including V₄R)

Left ventricular aneurysm

The development of a left ventricular aneurysm is a late complication of myocardial infarction, seen (to varying degrees) in around 10 per cent of survivors. The presence of an aneurysm can lead to persistent ST segment elevation in those chest leads that 'look at' the affected region (Fig. 9.9).

Ask the patient about a history of previous myocardial infarction and assess the patient for symptoms and signs related to the

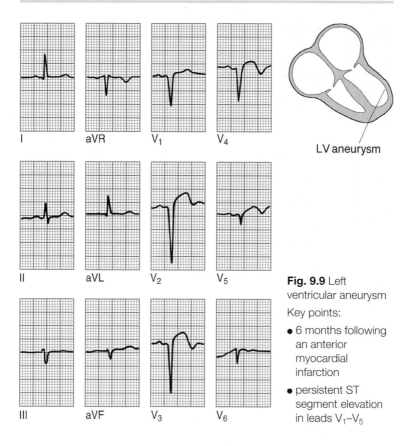

LV aneurysm

Fig. 9.9 Left ventricular aneurysm

Key points:

● 6 months following an anterior myocardial infarction
● persistent ST segment elevation in leads V_1–V_5

aneurysm itself. Aneurysms, being non-contractile, can lead to left ventricular dysfunction and thrombus formation. They can also be a focus for arrhythmia generation. Presenting symptoms can result from:

● heart failure
● embolic events
● arrhythmias.

The clinical signs of a left ventricular aneurysm are a 'double impulse' on precordial palpation and a fourth heart sound on auscultation. A chest X-ray may reveal a bulge on the cardiac outline. The investigation of choice is echocardiography, which will reveal the site of the aneurysm and the presence of mural thrombus, as well as allowing assessment of overall left ventricular function.

Patients with left ventricular aneurysms may benefit from treatment for heart failure and use of anticoagulation and anti-arrhythmic drugs. Consideration may also be given to surgical removal of the aneurysm (aneurysmectomy) or even cardiac transplantation where appropriate. Specialist referral is therefore recommended.

 SEEK HELP

A left ventricular aneurysm warrants specialist assessment. Obtain the advice of a cardiologist without delay.

Prinzmetal's (vasospastic) angina

Prinzmetal's angina refers to reversible myocardial ischaemia that results from coronary artery spasm. Although it can occur with normal coronary arteries, in over 90 per cent of cases the spasm is superimposed upon some degree of atherosclerosis. Although any artery can be affected, spasm most commonly occurs in the right coronary artery. During an episode of vasospasm, the patient develops ST segment elevation in the affected territory (Fig. 9.10).

Although the combination of chest pain and ST segment elevation often suggests myocardial infarction, vasospastic angina is distinguished by the transient nature of the ST segment elevation. Unlike myocardial infarction, the ECG changes of vasospastic angina resolve entirely when the episode of chest pain settles. Ask the patient about a history of prior episodes of chest pain, which typically occur at rest and particularly overnight in vasospastic angina. Patients may also have a history of other vasospastic disorders, such as Raynaud's phenomenon.

The ST segment elevation of vasospastic angina may be accompanied by tall 'hyperacute' T waves or, sometimes, T wave inversion. Transient intraventricular conduction defects, such as a bundle branch or fascicular block, can also occur.

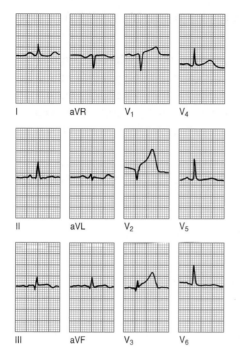

Fig. 9.10 Prinzmetal's (vasospastic) angina

Key point:

- anterior ST segment elevation during episode of chest pain

Treatment for vasospastic angina should include a calcium-channel blocker and/or a nitrate. Vasospastic angina can worsen with use of beta blockers, because they act on vasodilatory beta receptors while leaving vasoconstrictory alpha receptors unblocked.

Pericarditis

The ST segment elevation of pericarditis (Fig. 9.11) has four characteristics that, while not pathognomonic, help to distinguish it from acute myocardial infarction:

- The ST segment elevation is typically widespread, affecting all of those leads (anterolateral and inferior) that 'look at' the inflamed epicardium. Leads aVR and V_1 usually show reciprocal ST segment depression.
- The ST segment elevation is characteristically 'saddle shaped' (concave upward).

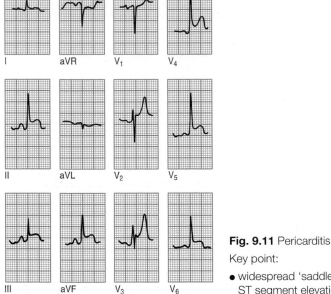

Fig. 9.11 Pericarditis

Key point:

- widespread 'saddle-shaped' ST segment elevation

- T wave inversion occurs only after the ST segments have returned to baseline.
- Q waves do not develop.

The assessment of a patient with pericarditis should aim not only at confirming the diagnosis but also at establishing the cause (Table 9.3).

Clinically, the pain of pericarditis can usually be distinguished from that of myocardial infarction. Although both produce a retrosternal pain, that of pericarditis is sharp and pleuritic, exacerbated by inspiration and relieved by sitting forward. A friction rub on auscultation is pathognomonic of pericarditis.

Direct treatment of the underlying cause should be carried out where possible. Anti-inflammatory agents (e.g. indomethacin) are often effective. Systemic corticosteroids are used in more

Table 9.3 Causes of pericarditis

- Infectious
  - viral (e.g. Coxsackie)
  - bacterial (e.g. *Staphylococcus*)
  - tuberculous
- Myocardial infarction (first few days)
- Dressler's syndrome (1 month or more post-myocardial infarction)
- Uraemia
- Malignancy
- Connective tissue disease
- Radiotherapy

difficult cases, although their role is controversial and they should not be considered without first obtaining specialist advice.

High take-off

Elevation of the ST segment is sometimes seen in the anterior chest leads as a variant of normal, and is referred to as 'high take-off' or 'early repolarization'. A high take-off ST segment always follows an S wave and is not associated with reciprocal ST segment depression; compare its appearances in Fig. 9.12 with the earlier ECGs in this chapter.

Whenever you suspect ST segment elevation to be just high take-off, always endeavour to find earlier ECGs for confirmation.

ARE THE ST SEGMENTS DEPRESSED?

Again, look carefully at the ST segment in each lead to see if it is isoelectric (on the same level as the ECG's baseline). If it is below this level, the ST segment is depressed.

If ST segment depression is present, think of the following possible causes:

- myocardial ischaemia
- acute posterior myocardial infarction

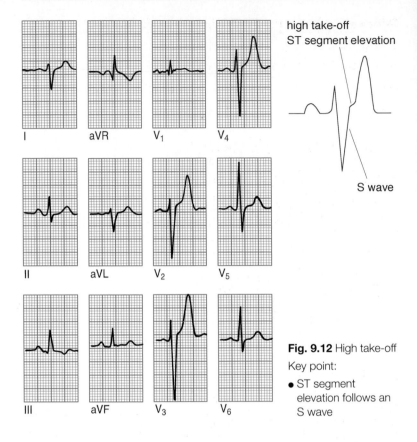

Fig. 9.12 High take-off

Key point:

- ST segment elevation follows an S wave

- drugs (e.g. digoxin, quinidine)
- ventricular hypertrophy with 'strain'.

If any of these is a possibility, turn to the following pages for guidance on what to do next.

Myocardial ischaemia

Unlike myocardial infarction, ischaemia is reversible and so the associated ECG abnormalities are seen only while the patient is experiencing an episode of pain. ST segment depression is the commonest abnormality associated with ischaemia and is usually 'horizontal' (cf. the 'reverse tick' with digoxin effect, p. 173).

Other changes seen in myocardial ischaemia include:

● T wave inversion (Chapter 10)
● T wave 'pseudonormalization' (Chapter 10).

Figure 9.13 shows the ECG of a patient with coronary artery disease during an episode of chest pain.

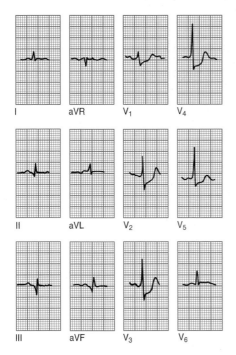

Fig. 9.13 Myocardial ischaemia
Key point:

● anterior ST segment
   depression with angina

If myocardial ischaemia is a possibility in your patient, ask about a history of angina and previous myocardial infarctions. Also ask about risk factors for coronary artery disease (see Table 9.1). Stable angina can be assessed further by exercise ECG testing (Chapter 16).

The management of stable angina includes:

● modifying any risk factors (e.g. smoking, hypertension)
● aspirin, 75 mg once daily
● glyceryl trinitrate sublingually as required.

Add in anti-anginal therapy as necessary to control symptoms:

- beta blocker
- calcium-channel blocker
- long-acting oral or transdermal or buccal nitrate
- nicorandil.

If anti-anginal drugs fail to control symptoms adequately, consider cardiac catheterization with a view to:

- percutaneous transluminal coronary angioplasty
- coronary artery bypass surgery.

Rapidly worsening chest pain, chest pain of recent onset or chest pain at rest indicates unstable angina or non-ST segment elevation acute coronary syndrome. This is a medical emergency, with a 1-year mortality of up to 20 per cent in untreated patients, so urgent treatment is essential. Initial treatment includes:

- bedrest
- analgesia
- aspirin
- beta blockers
- heparin
- intravenous nitrates
- a glycoprotein IIb/IIIa inhibitor (eptifibatide or tirofiban).

If unstable angina does not settle with drug treatment, consider cardiac catheterization with a view to urgent intervention – discuss this with a cardiologist.

 ACT QUICKLY

Unstable angina is a medical emergency. Prompt diagnosis and treatment are essential.

Acute posterior myocardial infarction

Acute posterior myocardial infarction is discussed in Chapter 8. It can cause ST segment depression in the chest leads V_1–V_3, together with:

● dominant R waves
● upright, tall T waves.

An example is shown in Fig. 8.4.

The management of posterior myocardial infarction is the same of that of other Q wave myocardial infarctions, as outlined earlier in this chapter.

 ACT QUICKLY

Acute myocardial infarction is a medical emergency. Prompt diagnosis and treatment are essential.

Drugs

Two anti-arrhythmic drugs affect the ST segment:

● digoxin
● quinidine.

Digoxin has a characteristic effect on the ST segment, which is just one of a number of its effects on the whole ECG (Table 9.4). The ST segment depression seen with digoxin is described as a 'reverse tick' and is most obvious in leads with tall R waves (Fig. 9.14).

You must always distinguish between digoxin effects, which may be apparent at therapeutic doses, and digoxin toxicity, which indicates overdosage. If digoxin toxicity is a possibility, ask about symptoms (anorexia, nausea, vomiting, abdominal pain and visual disturbance) and check the patient's digoxin and plasma potassium levels (arrhythmias are more likely if the patient is hypokalaemic).

Table 9.4 Effects of digoxin on the ECG

At therapeutic levels
- ST segment depression ('reverse tick')
- Reduction in T wave size
- Shortening of the QT interval

At toxic levels
- T wave inversion
- Arrhythmias – almost any, but especially:
  - sinus bradycardia
  - paroxysmal atrial tachycardia with block
  - atrioventricular block
  - ventricular ectopics
  - ventricular bigeminy
  - ventricular tachycardia

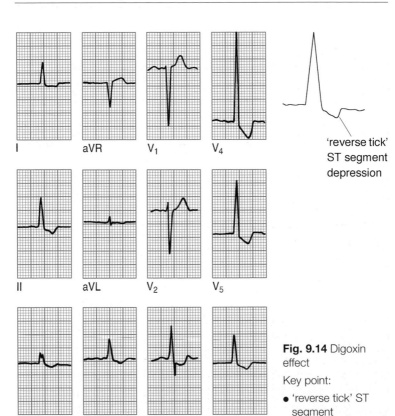

I   aVR   V₁   V₄

'reverse tick' ST segment depression

II   aVL   V₂   V₅

III   aVF   V₃   V₆

Fig. 9.14 Digoxin effect

Key point:
- 'reverse tick' ST segment depression

Treat digoxin toxicity by stopping the drug and, where necessary, correcting potassium levels and treating arrhythmias. A digoxin-specific antibody may be used if the problem is life threatening, but not without expert advice.

Quinidine also has a number of effects on the ECG, one of which is ST segment depression (which is not 'reverse tick' in character).

DRUG POINT

A complete drug history is essential in any patient with an abnormal ECG.

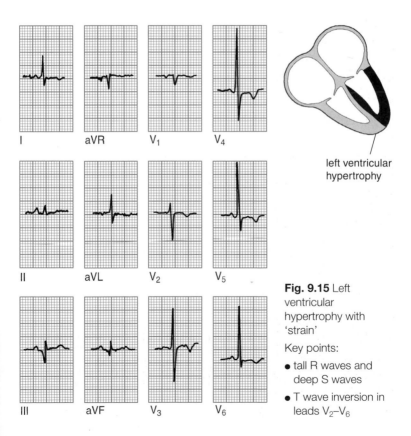

left ventricular hypertrophy

Fig. 9.15 Left ventricular hypertrophy with 'strain'

Key points:

- tall R waves and deep S waves

- T wave inversion in leads V_2–V_6

Ventricular hypertrophy with 'strain'

The appearances of both left and right ventricular hypertrophy are discussed in Chapter 8. The 'strain' pattern is said to be present when, in addition to tall R waves and deep S waves, there is also:

● ST segment depression
● T wave inversion

in the leads that 'look at' the affected ventricle (Fig. 9.15).

The term 'strain' is rather misleading, because the underlying mechanism is unclear. If you see T wave inversion in the presence of other ECG evidence of ventricular hypertrophy, assess the patient carefully as described in Chapter 8, both for further evidence of ventricular hypertrophy and for an underlying cause.

Summary

To assess the ST segment, ask the following questions:

1. Are the ST segments elevated?

If 'yes', consider:
● acute myocardial infarction
● left ventricular aneurysm
● Prinzmetal's (vasospastic) angina
● pericarditis
● high take-off.

2. Are the ST segments depressed?

If 'yes', consider:
● myocardial ischaemia
● acute posterior myocardial infarction
● drugs (digoxin, quinidine)
● ventricular hypertrophy with 'strain'.

10

THE T WAVE

After examining the ST segment, look carefully at the size and orientation of the T wave. The T wave corresponds to ventricular repolarization. The shape and orientation of normal T waves are shown in Fig. 10.1.

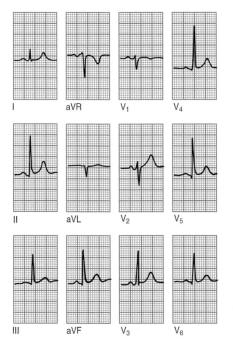

Fig. 10.1 Normal 12-lead ECG

Key point:

• T wave shape and orientation vary from lead to lead

It is normal for the T wave to be inverted in lead aVR. In some cases, T wave inversion can also be normal in leads III, V_1 and V_2, and these occurrences are discussed later in this chapter.

T waves can be abnormal in one of three ways, so the questions you need to ask about them are:

- Are the T waves too tall?
- Are the T waves too small?
- Are any of the T waves inverted?

ARE THE T WAVES TOO TALL?

There is no clearly defined normal range for T wave height, although, as a general guide, a T wave should be no more than half the size of the preceding QRS complex. Your ability to recognize abnormally tall T waves will improve as you examine increasing numbers of ECGs and gain experience of the normal variations that occur.

If you suspect that the T waves are abnormally tall, consider whether your patient could have either of the following:

- hyperkalaemia
- acute myocardial infarction.

If either is a possibility, turn to the following pages for guidance on what to do next.

Bear in mind, however, that tall T waves are often just a variant of normal, especially if you are judging just a single ECG. Your level of suspicion should be higher if you are comparing against earlier ECGs from the same patient and the height of the T waves has increased significantly.

Hyperkalaemia

An elevated plasma potassium level can cause tall 'tented' T waves (Fig. 10.2). Hyperkalaemia may also widen the T waves so that the entire ST segment is incorporated into the upstroke of the T wave. Hyperkalaemia may also cause:

- flattening and even loss of the P wave
- lengthening of the PR interval
- widening of the QRS complex
- arrhythmias.

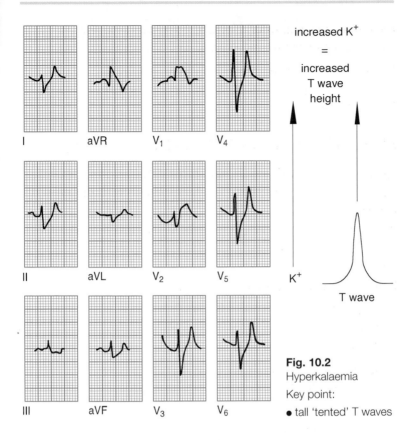

Fig. 10.2
Hyperkalaemia
Key point:
• tall 'tented' T waves

If the diagnosis is confirmed by an elevated plasma
potassium level, assess the patient for symptoms and
signs of an underlying cause (e.g. renal failure).
In particular, review their treatment chart for inappropriate
potassium supplements and potassium-sparing
diuretics.

 DRUG POINT

A complete drug history is essential in any patient with an
abnormal ECG.

Because of the risk of fatal cardiac arrhythmias, hyperkalaemia needs urgent treatment if it is causing ECG abnormalities or the plasma potassium level is above 6.5 mmol/L.

 ACT QUICKLY

Severe hyperkalaemia is a medical emergency. Prompt diagnosis and treatment are essential.

Acute myocardial infarction

Tall 'hyperacute' T waves, together with ST segment elevation, may be seen in the early stages of an acute myocardial infarction (Fig. 10.3). Increased T wave height may be a result of potassium released from damaged myocytes, leading to a localized hyperkalaemia.

Tall T waves are particularly characteristic of acute posterior myocardial infarction (p. 136). Infarction of the posterior wall of the left ventricle leads to reciprocal (i.e. 'mirror-image') changes when viewed from the perspective of the anterior chest leads. Thus, the usual myocardial infarction appearances of pathological Q waves, ST segment elevation and inverted T waves will appear as R waves, ST segment depression and upright, tall T waves when viewed from leads V_1–V_3 (see Fig. 8.4).

The diagnosis and management of acute myocardial infarction are discussed in detail on p. 156.

 SEEK HELP

Acute myocardial infarction requires urgent treatment. Obtain the advice of a cardiologist without delay.

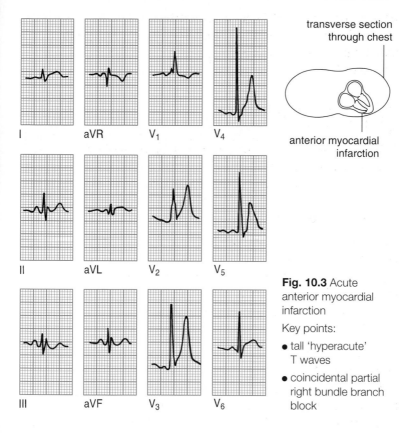

transverse section through chest

anterior myocardial infarction

Fig. 10.3 Acute anterior myocardial infarction

Key points:

- tall 'hyperacute' T waves
- coincidental partial right bundle branch block

ARE THE T WAVES TOO SMALL?

As with tall T waves, the judgement of whether T waves are abnormally small is subjective.

If you suspect that the T waves are abnormally small, consider whether your patient could have one of the following:

- hypokalaemia
- pericardial effusion
- hypothyroidism.

Advice about the diagnosis and treatment of each of these is given on the following pages.

Hypokalaemia

Just as hyperkalaemia causes tall T waves, so hypokalaemia causes small T waves (Fig. 10.4). Look carefully for other ECG changes that may accompany hypokalaemia:

- first-degree heart block
- depression of the ST segment
- prominent U waves.

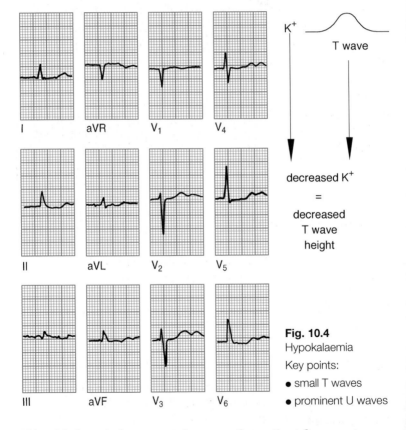

Fig. 10.4
Hypokalaemia
Key points:
- small T waves
- prominent U waves

If hypokalaemia is suspected, assess the patient for symptoms (e.g. muscle weakness, cramps) and review the treatment chart. Although a number of conditions lead to hypokalaemia, the commonest cause is diuretics.

DRUG POINT

A complete drug history is essential in any patient with an abnormal ECG.

Check the plasma electrolytes to confirm the diagnosis. Oral potassium supplements are sufficient if the plasma potassium level is above 2.5 mmol/L and the patient is asymptomatic. More severe hypokalaemia, or the presence of symptoms, requires cautious correction with a slow intravenous infusion of potassium chloride.

 ACT QUICKLY

Severe hypokalaemia is a medical emergency. Prompt diagnosis and treatment are essential.

Pericardial effusion

If the whole ECG, and not just the T waves, is of a low voltage, think about the possibility of pericardial effusion.

For a detailed discussion of the investigation and treatment of pericardial effusion, turn to p. 141.

Hypothyroidism

Hypothyroidism can cause small QRS complexes and small T waves, but the most characteristic finding is sinus bradycardia (p. 32).

Perform a careful history and examination, and confirm the diagnosis with T_3, T_4 and thyroid-stimulating hormone levels.

ARE ANY OF THE T WAVES INVERTED?

If T wave inversion is present, begin by asking:

● Could this be normal?

T wave inversion is considered normal in:

● leads aVR and V_1 (see Fig. 10.1)
● lead V_2 in younger people
● lead V_3 in black people (Fig. 10.5).

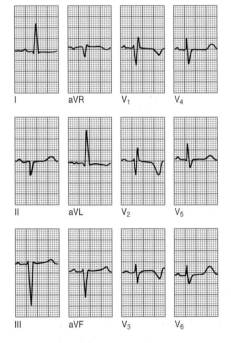

I	aVR	V_1	V_4
II	aVL	V_2	V_5
III	aVF	V_3	V_6

Fig. 10.5 T wave inversion in a normal black person

Key point:

● T wave inversion can be normal in leads V_1–V_3 in black people

T wave inversion in lead III can also be normal, and may be accompanied by a small Q wave – both of these findings can disappear if the ECG is repeated with the patient's breath held in inspiration (see Fig. 7.3).

T wave inversion in any other lead is generally considered abnormal, and if it is present, consider whether your patient has one of the following:

● myocardial ischaemia
● myocardial infarction
● ventricular hypertrophy with 'strain'
● digoxin toxicity.

You can find advice about the recognition and management of each of these conditions on the following pages.

There are also a number of conditions in which T wave inversion occurs in combination with other ECG abnormalities. If the ECG has been normal up to this point of the assessment, it is unlikely that any of the following are to blame for the T wave inversion. None the less, if you still have not found a cause after going through the list above, consider:

● repolarization abnormalities following a paroxysmal tachycardia (Chapter 3)
● bundle branch block (Chapter 8)
● pericarditis (Chapter 9)
● permanent ventricular pacing (Chapter 14).

Finally, there are four conditions in which T wave inversion can occur but the ECG is not diagnostic:

● hyperventilation
● mitral valve prolapse
● pulmonary embolism
● subarachnoid haemorrhage.

If your patient has one of these conditions, you do not need to look for another cause of T wave inversion unless there are other reasons to suspect one.

Myocardial ischaemia

ST segment depression is the commonest manifestation of myocardial ischaemia (Chapter 9), but T wave inversion may

also occur in the leads that 'look at' the affected areas
(Fig. 10.6). Because ischaemia is reversible, these ECG
abnormalities will only be observed during an ischaemic
episode.

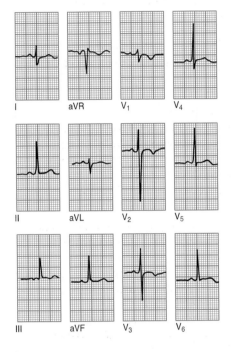

Fig. 10.6 T wave inversion with myocardial ischaemia

Key point:

- reversible T wave inversion (leads V_1–V_3) with myocardial ischaemia

Patients whose T waves are inverted to begin with (e.g.
following a myocardial infarction) may develop temporarily
upright T waves during ischaemic episodes. This is referred
to as T wave 'pseudonormalization'.

The management of myocardial ischaemia is described in detail
on p. 170.

Myocardial infarction

T wave inversion can occur not only as a temporary change
in myocardial ischaemia but also as a more prolonged (and
sometimes permanent) change in myocardial infarction.

In Chapter 9, we mentioned that myocardial infarctions are often divided into:

- Q wave infarcts or ST segment elevation myocardial infarction (STEMI)
- non-Q wave infarcts or non-ST segment elevation myocardial infarction (NSTEMI).

T wave inversion can occur in either type of infarct – the defining characteristic is whether or not Q waves appear.

Q wave vs non-Q wave infarction

The suggestion that Q wave infarcts always involve the *full thickness* of the myocardium, whereas non-Q wave infarcts only involve the *subendocardial* region, is misleading. Post-mortem studies have shown that this distinction is often incorrect, and so the terms 'full thickness' and 'subendocardial' are probably better avoided.

So why make the distinction between Q wave and non-Q wave infarcts at all? It is important for three reasons. First, there is currently no definitive evidence that thrombolysis improves prognosis in non-Q wave infarction. Second, patients with non-Q wave infarction may be at higher risk of re-infarction than those presenting with Q wave infarcts, although there is no overall difference in 3-year mortality. Third, there is some evidence that glycoprotein IIb/IIIa inhibitors may be of benefit in selected patients with NSTEMI.

In Q wave infarction, the T wave inversion accompanies the return of the elevated ST segment to baseline (Fig. 10.7). T wave inversion may be permanent, or the T wave may return to normal.

Non-Q wave infarction also causes T wave inversion (Fig. 10.8), although it can also manifest as ST segment depression alone.

If you see abnormal T wave inversion on an ECG, question the patient about any history of chest pain and

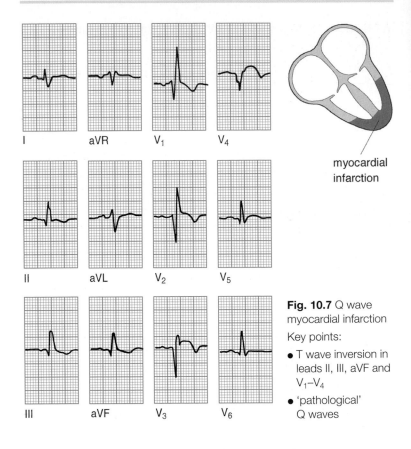

Fig. 10.7 Q wave myocardial infarction

Key points:

- T wave inversion in leads II, III, aVF and V_1–V_4
- 'pathological' Q waves

previous angina or myocardial infarctions and assess their risk factors for ischaemic heart disease (see Table 9.1).

The management of Q wave myocardial infarction is detailed in Chapter 9.

 ACT QUICKLY

Acute myocardial infarction is a medical emergency. Prompt diagnosis and treatment are essential.

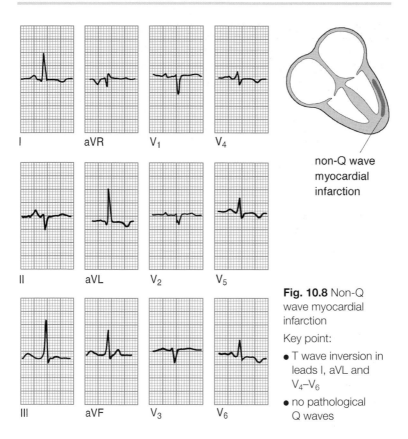

I aVR V₁ V₄

II aVL V₂ V₅

III aVF V₃ V₆

non-Q wave
myocardial
infarction

Fig. 10.8 Non-Q
wave myocardial
infarction

Key point:

- T wave inversion in
  leads I, aVL and
  V_4–V_6

- no pathological
  Q waves

Ventricular hypertrophy

In addition to tall R waves and deep S waves (Chapter 8),
ventricular hypertrophy can also cause ST segment depression
and T wave inversion. This is commonly referred to as a
'strain' pattern (p. 176).

If present, the 'strain' pattern is seen in the leads that 'look at'
the hypertrophied ventricle. With left ventricular hypertrophy
the abnormalities will be seen in leads I, aVL and V_4–V_6. Right
ventricular hypertrophy causes changes in leads V_1–V_3.

The term 'strain' is rather misleading because the
underlying mechanism is unclear. Although some conditions,

such as massive pulmonary embolism, can certainly place a ventricle under an increased workload and are associated with the 'strain' pattern, it is also seen in cases of ventricular hypertrophy where there is no apparent stress on the ventricle.

If you see T wave inversion in the presence of other ECG evidence of ventricular hypertrophy, assess the patient carefully as described in Chapter 8.

Digoxin toxicity

Always check if a patient with T wave inversion is receiving treatment with digoxin, as this can be an indication of digoxin toxicity (Fig. 10.9). This is just one of a number of ECG changes that can be seen in patients taking digoxin (see Table 9.4).

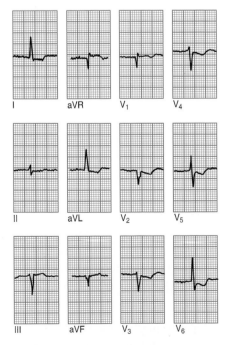

Fig. 10.9 Digoxin toxicity

Key points:

- T wave inversion in leads V_2–V_6
- patient on digoxin for atrial fibrillation

The diagnosis and treatment of digoxin toxicity are covered in more detail on p. 173.

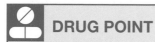

DRUG POINT

A complete drug history is essential in any patient with an abnormal ECG.

Summary

To assess the T wave, ask the following questions:

1. Are the T waves too tall?

If 'yes', consider:
- hyperkalaemia
- acute myocardial infarction.

2. Are the T waves too small?

If 'yes', consider:
- hypokalaemia
- pericardial effusion
- hypothyroidism.

3. Are any of the T waves inverted?

If 'yes', consider:
- normal (leads aVR and V_1)
- normal variant (leads V_2, V_3 and III)
- myocardial ischaemia
- myocardial infarction
- ventricular hypertrophy with 'strain'
- digoxin toxicity.

Also bear in mind:
- repolarization abnormalities following a paroxysmal tachycardia (Chapter 3)
- bundle branch block (Chapter 8)
- pericarditis (Chapter 9)
- permanent ventricular pacing (Chapter 14)
- hyperventilation
- mitral valve prolapse
- pulmonary embolism
- subarachnoid haemorrhage.

THE QT INTERVAL

A fter examining the T waves, measure the QT interval. This is the time from the *start* of the QRS complex to the *end* of the T wave (Fig. 11.1), and it represents the total duration of electrical activity (depolarization and repolarization) in the ventricles.

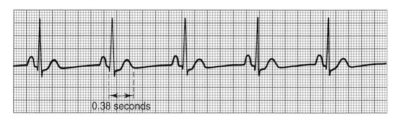

0.38 seconds

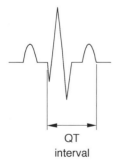

Fig. 11.1 The QT interval

QT interval

Key point:

● QT interval is 0.38 s in this patient

When determining the duration of the QT interval, it is important to measure it to the end of the T wave and not the U wave (if one is present – see Chapter 12). Mistaking a U wave for a T wave is easily done and overestimates the QT interval. To reduce the likelihood of this, measure the QT interval in lead aVL, where U waves are least prominent.

As with any interval in the ECG, there are only two possible abnormalities of the QT interval:

● The QT interval can be too long.
● The QT interval can be too short.

Unfortunately, deciding whether or not the QT interval is normal is not entirely straightforward, because the duration varies according to the patient's heart rate: the faster the heart rate, the shorter the QT interval. To allow for this, you must calculate the corrected QT interval (QT$_c$) using the following formula:

$$QT_c = \frac{QT}{\sqrt{RR}}$$

where QT$_c$ is the corrected QT interval, QT is the measured QT interval and RR is the measured RR interval (all measurements in seconds).

If you are interested in the theory behind QT interval correction, read the box below.

A normal QT$_c$ interval is 0.35–0.43 s long. When you assess the QT interval, therefore, ask yourself the following two questions:

● Is the QT$_c$ interval shorter than 0.35 s?
● Is the QT$_c$ interval longer than 0.43 s?

If the answer to either question is 'yes', turn to the relevant section of this chapter to find out what to do next. If 'no', you can move on to the next chapter.

Why correct the QT interval?

Correction of the QT interval is necessary because the normal QT interval varies with heart rate: the faster the heart rate, the shorter the normal QT interval. Although graphs and tables of normal QT intervals at different heart rates are available, it is inconvenient to have to look up the normal range every time you want to check someone's QT interval.

A much better way to assess a QT interval is to correct it to what it *would* be if the patient's heart rate was 60 beats/min. By doing this, all you will then need to remember is *one* normal range for the QT interval.

You will need a pocket calculator to calculate the corrected QT interval ('QT_c interval'). Divide the patient's measured QT interval (measured in seconds) by the square root of their RR interval (also measured in seconds). This is Bazett's formula:

$$QT_c = \frac{QT}{\sqrt{RR}}$$

The RR interval is the time between consecutive R waves, and can be either measured directly from the ECG or calculated by dividing 60 by the patient's heart rate. For example, at a heart rate of 80 beats/min the RR interval is 0.75 s.

Many of the more sophisticated ECG machines automatically print out a value for the QT_c interval on the ECG. However, always check for yourself values that are automatically measured in this way, as errors do occur.

The normal range for the QT interval at a heart rate of 60 beats/min, and thus for the QT_c interval, is 0.35–0.43 s.

IS THE QT_C INTERVAL SHORTER THAN 0.35 SECONDS?

If the answer is 'yes', your patient's corrected QT interval is shorter than normal and you should check for the following:

- hypercalcaemia
- digoxin effect.

If either of these is a possibility, read the following pages to find out what to do next.

Shortening of the QT_c interval is also recognized in hyperthermia.

Having established the diagnosis of hyperthermia clinically, you will not need to look for another cause for a shortened QT_c interval unless there is a good reason to do so.

Hypercalcaemia

The shortened QT interval in hypercalcaemia results from abnormally rapid ventricular repolarization (Fig. 11.2).

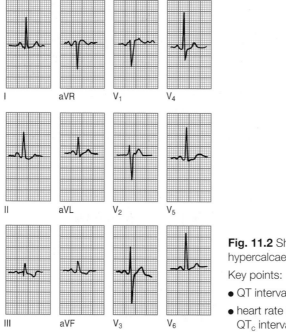

Fig. 11.2 Short QT interval in hypercalcaemia

Key points:

• QT interval is 0.26 s

• heart rate is 100 beats/min, QT_c interval is 0.34 s

Symptoms of hypercalcaemia include anorexia, weight loss, nausea, vomiting, abdominal pain, constipation, polydipsia, polyuria, weakness and depression.

A prominent U wave may also be seen in hypercalcaemia. Confirm the diagnosis with a plasma calcium level (correcting the result for the patient's current albumin level). The underlying causes that you need to consider are listed in Table 11.1.

Table 11.1 Causes of hypercalcaemia

- Hyperparathyroidism
  - primary
  - tertiary
- Malignancy (including myeloma)
- Drugs
  - thiazide diuretics
  - excessive vitamin D intake
- Sarcoidosis
- Thyrotoxicosis
- Milk-alkali syndrome

The treatment of hypercalcaemia depends, in the long term, on the underlying cause. Immediate management depends upon the symptoms and plasma calcium level. There is a risk of cardiac arrest with severe hypercalcaemia, so prompt recognition and treatment are essential.

Severe symptoms (e.g. vomiting, drowsiness) or a plasma calcium level greater than 3.5 mmol/L warrant urgent treatment as follows:

- intravenous 0.9% saline (e.g. 3–4 litres per 24 h)
- intravenous frusemide (20–40 mg every 6–12 h *after rehydration*)
- bisphosphonates (e.g. disodium pamidronate – single infusion of 30 mg over 2 h)
- discontinue thiazides/vitamin D compounds
- monitor urea and electrolytes and calcium levels every 12 h.

 ACT QUICKLY

Severe hypercalcaemia is a medical emergency. Prompt diagnosis and treatment are essential.

Digoxin effect

Shortening of the QT interval is one of several effects that treatment with digoxin has on the ECG (see Table 9.4).

It is important to note that digoxin *effects* are normal, and do not imply that the patient has digoxin *toxicity*. The effects of digoxin on the ECG are covered in more detail in Chapter 9.

 DRUG POINT

A complete drug history is essential in any patient with an abnormal ECG.

IS THE QT$_C$ INTERVAL LONGER THAN 0.43 SECONDS?

If the answer is 'yes', your patient's corrected QT interval is prolonged. The causes you need to consider are:

- hypocalcaemia
- drug effects
- acute myocarditis
- hereditary syndromes.

If any of these is a possibility, consult the following pages to find out what to do next.

In addition, there are also several conditions in which QT interval prolongation is recognized, but in which this abnormality is an interesting feature rather than a useful diagnostic pointer. Such conditions include:

- acute myocardial infarction
- cerebral injury
- hypertrophic cardiomyopathy
- hypothermia.

You simply need to be aware that QT interval prolongation is recognized in these conditions, so that you do not need to look for another cause unless clinically suspected.

Hypocalcaemia

Hypocalcaemia is a well-recognized cause of QT interval prolongation (Fig. 11.3).

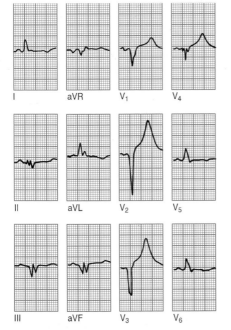

| I | aVR | V₁ | V₄ |

| II | aVL | V₂ | V₅ |

| III | aVF | V₃ | V₆ |

Fig. 11.3 Long QT interval in hypocalcaemia

Key points:

- QT interval is 0.57 s
- heart rate is 51 beats/min, QT$_c$ interval is 0.52 s

The clinical features (peripheral and circumoral paraesthesiae, tetany, fits and psychiatric disturbance) are characteristic. Look for Trousseau's sign (carpal spasm when the brachial artery is occluded with a blood-pressure cuff), Chvostek's sign (twitching of facial muscles when tapping over the facial nerve) and papilloedema. Confirm the diagnosis by checking a plasma calcium level on an uncuffed blood sample, not forgetting to check a simultaneous albumin level so that any necessary correction can be made.

Once a diagnosis of hypocalcaemia has been made, always look for the underlying cause (Table 11.2).

Table 11.2 Causes of hypocalcaemia

- Hypoparathyroidism
  - following thyroid surgery
  - autoimmune
  - congenital (DiGeorge syndrome)
- Pseudohypoparathyroidism
- Chronic renal failure
- Vitamin D deficiency/resistance
- Drugs (e.g. calcitonin)
- Acute pancreatitis

The treatment of hypocalcaemia depends upon the severity of symptoms. Treat severe hypocalcaemia with intravenous calcium (given as 10 mL calcium gluconate 10%). Treat those who have milder symptoms with oral calcium supplements and, if necessary, oral vitamin D derivatives. Carefully monitor plasma calcium levels to avoid overtreatment and consequent hypercalcaemia.

Drug effects

A number of anti-arrhythmic drugs cause prolongation of the QT interval by slowing myocardial conduction, and thus repolarization. Examples include quinidine, procainamide and flecainide. QT interval prolongation is also seen with tricyclic antidepressants.

Drug-induced QT interval prolongation is associated with torsades de pointes (Chapter 3), which can lead to ventricular fibrillation and sudden cardiac death. The problem therefore requires immediate attention, and referral to a cardiologist for review of anti-arrhythmic drug treatment is recommended.

 DRUG POINT

A complete drug history is essential in any patient with an abnormal ECG.

Acute myocarditis

QT interval prolongation can occur with any cause of acute myocarditis, although it is usually associated with rheumatoid carditis.

Presenting features often include a fever, chest discomfort, palpitations and symptoms of heart failure (dyspnoea and fatigue). Examination may reveal quiet heart sounds, a friction rub, tachycardia, a fourth heart sound and gallop rhythm. There may also be features specific to the underlying cause (Table 11.3).

Table 11.3 Causes of myocarditis

- Infectious
  - viral (e.g. Coxsackie, influenza)
  - bacterial (e.g. acute rheumatic fever, diphtheria)
  - protozoal (e.g. Chagas' disease, toxoplasmosis)
  - rickettsial
- Drug induced (e.g. chloroquine)
- Toxic agents (e.g. lead)
- Peripartum

Other ECG changes may be present, including:

- ST segment changes
- T wave inversion
- heart block (of any degree of severity)
- arrhythmias.

A chest X-ray may show cardiomegaly. A cardiac biopsy reveals acute inflammatory changes, and the levels of cardiac enzymes will be raised. Rarely, viral serology may establish the aetiology.

The treatment of acute myocarditis is supportive. Bedrest is recommended. Treat heart failure, arrhythmias and heart block as necessary. Antibiotics are indicated where a responsive organism is suspected. Although many patients will go on to make a good recovery, some are left with heart failure.

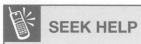

SEEK HELP

Acute myocarditis requires specialist assessment. Obtain the advice of a cardiologist without delay.

Hereditary syndromes

Prolongation of the QT interval occurs in two hereditary syndromes:

● Jervill and Lange–Nielsen syndrome
● Romano–Ward syndrome.

The autosomal recessive Jervill and Lange–Nielsen syndrome consists of congenital high-tone deafness, recurrent syncopal attacks and sudden death secondary to ventricular tachycardia, torsades de pointes and ventricular fibrillation. The arrhythmias are often triggered by exercise or stress.

The autosomal dominant Romano–Ward syndrome carries the same risk of ventricular arrhythmias but hearing is normal.

Prolonged QT intervals may be detected incidentally on an ECG in an asymptomatic individual, or in a patient presenting with a ventricular arrhythmia. Although rare, both syndromes are associated with torsades de pointes (Chapter 3) and sudden cardiac death. Referral to a cardiologist is recommended.

SEEK HELP

Hereditary long-QT syndromes are life threatening. Obtain the advice of a cardiologist without delay.

Summary

To assess the QT interval, ask the following questions:

1. Is the QT_c interval shorter than 0.35 s?

If 'yes', consider:
- hypercalcaemia
- digoxin effect (p. 173).

Also bear in mind:
- hyperthermia.

2. Is the QT_c interval longer than 0.43 s?

If 'yes', consider:
- hypocalcaemia
- drug effects
- acute myocarditis
- hereditary syndromes.

Also bear in mind:
- acute myocardial infarction (p. 156)
- cerebral injury
- hypertrophic cardiomyopathy
- hypothermia.

12

THE U WAVE

The U wave follows the T wave (Fig. 12.1) and is commonly seen in normal ECGs, although it can be difficult to discern clearly. When present, U waves are most clearly seen in the anterior chest leads V_2–V_4.

Although it is suggested that the U wave is caused by repolarization of the interventricular septum, this is by no means certain.

Normally, U waves are small and point in the same direction as the preceding T wave. Therefore, inverted U waves usually follow inverted T waves, and result from the same clinical abnormality (see Chapter 10).

U waves can also be abnormal in their own right, so when you assess the U wave, ask the following question:

● Do the U waves appear too prominent?

If the answer is 'yes', you will find a list of causes to consider in the next section.

DO THE U WAVES APPEAR TOO PROMINENT?

This is not a straightforward question to answer, because there is no normal range that you can apply to the height of a U wave. Suspecting the U waves are too prominent therefore depends upon subjective judgement rather than an objective measurement, and there is no substitute for reporting large

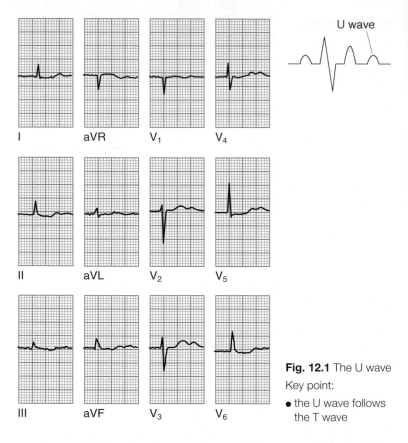

Fig. 12.1 The U wave

Key point:

- the U wave follows the T wave

numbers of ECGs to gain experience of the range of normality of the U wave (and, for that matter, all other aspects of the ECG).

It follows on from this that you should not attach too much weight to U wave prominence. Simply regard it as a clue that your patient may have one of the following:

- hypokalaemia
- hypercalcaemia
- hyperthyroidism.

If any of these is a possibility, turn to the appropriate section of this chapter to find out what to do next.

Hypokalaemia

Prominent U waves can be just one of a number of ECG abnormalities seen in the hypokalaemic patient (Fig. 12.2). Other associated ECG changes include:

● first-degree atrioventricular block (Chapter 6)
● depression of the ST segment (Chapter 9)
● small T waves (Chapter 10).

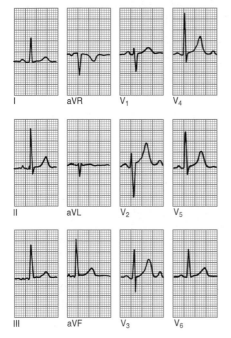

Fig. 12.2 Hypokalaemia
Key point:

● prominent U waves in leads V_2–V_4

The investigation and treatment of hypokalaemia are discussed in detail on p. 182.

 ACT QUICKLY

Severe hypokalaemia is a medical emergency. Prompt diagnosis and treatment are essential.

Hypercalcaemia

Always think of hypercalcaemia if you see prominent U waves, although hypercalcaemia is more characteristically associated with shortening of the QT interval (Chapter 11).

Confirm the diagnosis with a plasma calcium level (correcting the result for the patient's current albumin level).

The management of hypercalcaemia is discussed in detail on p. 196.

Hyperthyroidism

Prominent U waves in association with a tachycardia (Chapter 2) should prompt you to think of hyperthyroidism, although the U wave abnormality is not commonly seen in this condition.

Confirm the diagnosis with T_3, T_4 and thyroid-stimulating hormone levels.

Summary

To assess the U wave, ask the following question:

1. Do the U waves appear too prominent?

If 'yes', consider:
- hypokalaemia
- hypercalcaemia
- hyperthyroidism.

Note. U waves can also be inverted, but this usually accompanies T wave inversion, the causes of which are discussed in Chapter 10.

13

ARTEFACTS ON THE ECG

If you encounter ECG abnormalities that appear atypical or that do not fit with the patient's clinical condition, always consider the possibility that they may be artefacts caused by:

- electrode misplacement
- external electrical interference
- incorrect calibration
- incorrect paper speed
- patient movement.

Examples of each of these are discussed on the following pages.

Remember
- Never give undue weight to a single investigation, particularly if the result does not fit with your clinical findings.
- Do not hesitate to repeat an ECG if you suspect that the abnormalities could be artefacts.

ELECTRODE MISPLACEMENT

How to position each recording electrode correctly is discussed in Chapter 1. It can be quite easy to swap two electrodes over inadvertently, and this is particularly common with the limb electrodes.

Figure 13.1 shows an ECG recorded with the two arm electrodes swapped over. The abnormalities can be quite subtle, but you should always think of electrode misplacement if you see unexpected wave inversions.

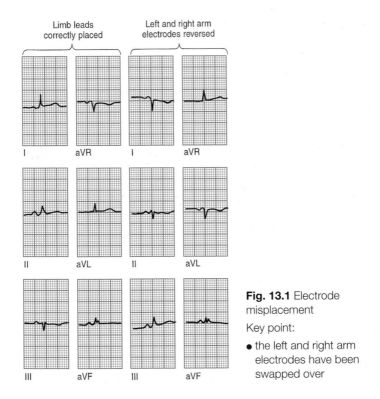

Fig. 13.1 Electrode misplacement

Key point:

- the left and right arm electrodes have been swapped over

EXTERNAL ELECTRICAL INTERFERENCE

External electrical interference (e.g. from electrical appliances) seldom causes difficulties when recording ECGs in hospital. However, for general practitioners who sometimes record ECGs in patients' homes, 50-Hz electrical interference from domestic appliances has been reported as a significant cause of ECG artefact, and this can make the ECG difficult or even impossible to interpret correctly.

Always bear this in mind when interpreting an ECG recorded in a patient's home. Unless the source of the interference can be identified and removed, there is little that can be done apart from repeating the recording with the patient in a new location.

INCORRECT CALIBRATION

The standard ECG is recorded so that a voltage of 1 mV makes the recording needle move 10 mm. Every ECG must include a calibration mark (Fig. 13.2) so that the gain setting can be checked.

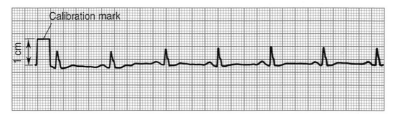

Fig. 13.2 Correct calibration

Key points: • note 1-cm calibration mark

  • 1 mV = 1 cm

Sometimes it is necessary to alter the gain setting, particularly if the QRS complexes are so big at the standard setting that they will not fit clearly on the paper. If it is necessary to change to a non-standard calibration, it is good practice to record this clearly by writing a note on the ECG. If you see waves that appear too big or too small, always double-check the size of the calibration mark (Fig. 13.3).

INCORRECT PAPER SPEED

In the UK and USA, the standard ECG recording speed is 25 mm/s, so that 1 small (1 mm) square equals 0.04 s. If the paper is run at double the speed (50 mm/s, which is standard in some parts of Europe), the waves will double in width

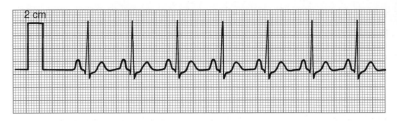

Fig. 13.3 Incorrect calibration
Key point: • 1 mV = 2 cm

(Fig. 13.4). Always label every ECG you record with the paper speed used and, if you use a non-standard setting, it is good practice to document this clearly at the top of the ECG.

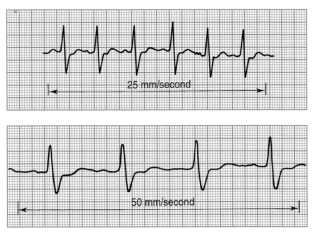

Fig. 13.4 Incorrect paper speed
Key point: • waves are abnormally wide at higher paper speeds

PATIENT MOVEMENT

The ECG records the electrical activity of the heart, but this is not the only source of electrical activity in the body. Skeletal muscle activity is also picked up on the ECG, and it is important for patients to lie still and relaxed while their ECGs are recorded. Unfortunately, this is not always possible, particularly if the patient is:

- uncooperative or agitated
- in respiratory distress
- suffering from a movement disorder.

Skeletal muscle activity is unavoidable during exercise testing. The use of signal-averaged ECGs, which 'average out' random electrical artefacts by combining a number of PQRST complexes, can help (Fig. 13.5). However, signal-averaged recordings can also be misleading by introducing artefactual changes of their own, and such recordings should always be interpreted with discretion.

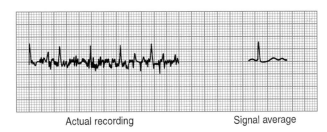

Actual recording   Signal average

Fig. 13.5 Signal-averaged ECG
Key point: ● electrical artefacts are reduced by signal averaging

Summary

For any ECG abnormality, always ask yourself:

1. Could this be artefactual?

If 'yes', consider:
- electrode misplacement
- external electrical interference
- incorrect calibration
- incorrect paper speed
- patient movement.

14

PACEMAKERS
AND AICDs

It is beyond the scope of this handbook to provide a detailed discussion of pacemakers and automatic implantable cardioverter defibrillators (AICDs). However, we have included a brief overview in this chapter for two reasons:

- Pacemakers and AICDs are effective treatments for a number of the problems described in this book.
- Pacing affects the appearance of the ECG.

On the following pages you will find a general description of what pacemakers and AICDs do, together with their indications.

WHAT DO PACEMAKERS DO?

Rapid advances in pacemaker technology have led to a remarkable increase in pacemaker sophistication, such that a wide range of different functions is now available. The most basic function of a pacemaker is to provide a 'safety net' for patients at risk of bradycardia. However, pacemakers that can terminate tachycardias are also available.

Pacemakers can either be **temporary**, to provide pacing in an emergency, or to tide patients over a short period of bradycardia (e.g. during a myocardial infarction) or until a permanent pacemaker can be implanted; or they can be

permanent, in which case the battery, electronics and electrode(s) are all implanted within the patient. Temporary pacemakers are usually transvenous, but transoesophageal and transcutaneous pacing can also be used.

Patients seldom need pacing all the time, so both temporary and permanent pacemakers can be set up to monitor the heart's activity and only provide impulses when necessary. In the case of permanent pacemakers, this is an effective way of prolonging the lifetime of the battery, typically to between 7 and 15 years.

Percussion pacing

Cardiac pacing can sometimes be achieved with no mechanical aids whatsoever. The technique of **percussion pacing** was first described in the 1960s and can help to maintain a good cardiac output in a bradycardic patient with considerably less trauma than chest compression. Percussion pacing is performed by delivering gentle blows to the precordium (alongside the lower left sternal edge) to stimulate QRS complexes – the technique can be remarkably effective and can buy enough time to arrange further treatment as appropriate.

INDICATIONS FOR TEMPORARY PACING

Patients awaiting permanent pacing

If patients have a severely symptomatic bradycardia but permanent pacing cannot be undertaken within an acceptable time, temporary pacing may be used to support them in the interim.

Acute myocardial infarction

In acute **inferior** myocardial infarction, damage to the artery that supplies the atrioventricular (AV) node can cause complete heart block and bradycardia. Few patients need help with temporary pacing, as blood pressure is usually maintained despite the slow heart rate. Temporary pacing is needed in second-degree and third-degree AV block with symptoms or haemodynamic disturbance.

Acute **anterior** myocardial infarction often causes hypotension as a result of damage to the left ventricle. Extensive infarction may involve the bundle branches in the interventricular septum and cause bradycardia. Mortality is high. Temporary pacing and inotropic support are necessary for second-degree and third-degree AV block, even when the condition is asymptomatic.

Tachycardia

Some tachycardias (including AV re-entry tachycardia and ventricular tachycardia) can be terminated by **overdrive pacing**. This should only be undertaken under the guidance of someone experienced in the technique – contact a cardiologist for assistance.

Perioperative pacing

See p. 221 for further information.

TEMPORARY PACEMAKER INSERTION AND CARE

Once the decision to insert a temporary pacemaker has been made, you must ensure that:

- the pacing wire is inserted using aseptic technique by a trained member of staff
- X-ray screening time is kept to a minimum
- a 'breathable' dressing is applied to the wound
- a chest X-ray is ordered (and looked at!) after the pacemaker insertion to check for pneumothorax
- the function of the pacemaker is monitored daily by checking the pacing threshold and ensuring the output is set at double the threshold
- the pacing wire does not become dislodged

- the pacing wire is removed at the earliest opportunity to prevent infection
- the pacing wire is replaced, if still required, after 5 days, after which time infection risk increases sharply
- temporary pacing is not withheld in acute myocardial infarction because of thrombolysis (the external jugular, brachiocephalic or femoral veins can be used for intravenous access routes in these circumstances, as these are superficial and easily compressed to control bleeding).

INDICATIONS FOR PERMANENT PACING

The decision to implant a *permanent* pacemaker must be made by a cardiologist, and you should seek their advice if you are uncertain about referring a patient. Generally speaking, the following are indications for a permanent pacemaker.

- **Third-degree AV block** with an episode of syncope or presyncope. Asymptomatic patients with acquired third-degree AV block and a ventricular rate less than 40 beats/min, or pauses greater than 3 s, should also be considered for pacing for prognostic reasons. Those with congenital third-degree AV block generally do not require pacing if they are asymptomatic, although they must be kept under regular review.
- **Second-degree AV block**, regardless of whether it is Mobitz type I or II, with an episode of symptomatic bradycardia.
- **Bifascicular** or **trifascicular block** with a clear history of syncope, or documented intermittent failure of the remaining fascicle.
- **Sick sinus syndrome** causing symptomatic bradycardia. Pacing is not usually necessary for asymptomatic patients.
- **Malignant vasovagal syndrome** is helped by pacing only if it is of the 'cardio-inhibitory' variety that causes a bradycardia.
- **Carotid sinus syndrome** is also only helped by pacing when it is of the cardio-inhibitory variety associated with a bradycardia.

SELECTION OF A PERMANENT PACEMAKER

A wide choice of permanent pacemakers is now available, each offering a different pacing strategy. The cardiologist will be responsible for selecting the most appropriate type of unit to be inserted, as well as for providing long-term follow-up.

There is an internationally accepted code of up to five letters to describe the type of pacemaker. Each letter describes an aspect of the pacemaker's function, as outlined in Table 14.1.

Table 14.1 Pacemaker codes

Letter	Refers to	Code	Meaning
1	Chamber(s) paced	A	Atrium
		V	Ventricle
		D	Dual (both chambers)
2	Chamber(s) sensed	A	Atrium
		V	Ventricle
		D	Dual (both chambers)
		O	None
3	Response to sensing	I	Inhibition of pacemaker
		T	Triggering of pacemaker
		D	Inhibition or triggering
		O	None
4	Rate response	R	Rate-responsive pacemaker
5	Anti-tachycardia functions	P	Pacing of tachycardias
		S	Shock delivered
		D	Dual (pacing and shock)
		O	None

The following are some of the most commonly encountered pacemakers.

- **VVI**: this pacemaker has a single lead that senses activity in the ventricle. If no activity is detected, the pacemaker will take over control of the rhythm by pacing the ventricle via the same lead.
- **AAI**: this pacemaker also has a single lead, which is implanted in the atrium. It monitors atrial (P wave) activity.

If normal atrial activity is not detected, it takes over by pacing the atria.

● **DDD**: this system has leads in both the atrium and the ventricle ('dual chamber'). It can both sense and pace via either lead. If it senses atrial activity but no ventricular activity, it will start pacing the ventricles in sequence with the atria. It can also pace the atria alone or, if AV conduction is blocked, pace the atria and ventricles sequentially.

● **AAIR, VVIR and DDDR**: the 'R' indicates that the pacemaker is rate responsive (see box below).

Rate responsiveness

A rate-responsive pacemaker adjusts its pacing rate according to the patient's level of activity to mimic the physiological response to exercise. There are several parameters that can be monitored by pacemakers to determine the patient's level of activity, including vibration, respiration and blood temperature.

PACING AND THE ECG

Pacemakers activate depolarization with electrical impulses, and these appear as pacing 'spikes' on the ECG (Fig. 14.1). In ventricular pacing, a pacing spike will be followed by a broad QRS complex (because the depolarization is not conducted by the normal, fast-conduction pathways).

When the atria are being paced via an atrial lead, the pacing spike will be followed by a P wave. This may be conducted normally via the AV junction and followed by a normal QRS complex. Alternatively, in dual-chamber sequential pacing, the P wave will be followed by a pacing spike from the ventricular lead and a broad QRS complex (Fig. 14.2).

Failure of a pacing spike to be followed by depolarization indicates a problem with 'capture', and a cardiologist should be contacted to arrange a pacemaker check.

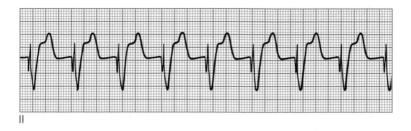

II

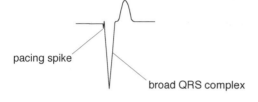

pacing spike

broad QRS complex

Fig. 14.1 Ventricular pacing

Key point:

● ventricular pacing spikes are followed by broad QRS complexes

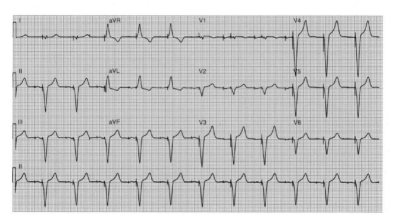

Fig. 14.2 Dual-chamber sequential pacing

Key points: ● atrial pacing spikes (small) are followed by P waves

● ventricular pacing spikes (large) are followed by broad QRS complexes

PACEMAKERS AND SURGERY

Pacemakers are relevant in surgery for two reasons:

● permanent pacemakers and diathermy
● temporary prophylactic perioperative pacing.

Surgeons and anaesthetists must always be made aware if a patient undergoing surgery has a permanent pacemaker. Always ascertain the pacemaker type (patients usually carry an identification card with the pacemaker code on it) and the original indication for its insertion. It may also be advisable to arrange a check of the pacemaker before and after surgery.

Particular care must be taken during the operation to avoid interference with, or damage to, the pacemaker from diathermy. A particular risk of diathermy is that of inappropriate pacemaker inhibition, causing bradycardia or even asystole; it is therefore important to monitor the patient's ventricular rate closely throughout the procedure. To minimize the dangers, place the active diathermy electrode at least 15 cm from the pacemaker's generator box, and the indifferent electrode as far from the box as possible.

Patients with certain cardiac conduction disorders who do *not* have a permanent pacemaker should be considered for a temporary pacemaker if they are about to undergo general anaesthesia. Temporary pacing is indicated in:

- third-degree AV block
- second-degree AV block.

Pacing is not usually necessary for bifascicular block unless the patient has a history of presyncope or syncope. Consult a cardiologist for further guidance.

AICDs

AICDs have proved to be invaluable in the management of life-threatening ventricular arrhythmias. AICDs are only a little larger than permanent pacemakers and are implanted subcutaneously, usually in the same location as permanent pacemakers, although some of the older, bigger, units were implanted abdominally.

AICDs continually monitor the cardiac rhythm looking for ventricular arrhythmias. If an episode of ventricular tachycardia occurs, the device will normally start by trying to overdrive pace the arrhythmia to try to terminate it. If that fails, the device will usually go on to deliver a shock. If ventricular fibrillation is detected, a shock is delivered as first-line therapy. The parameters by which AICDs diagnose arrhythmias and respond to them can be individually programmed into the device after it has been implanted, so that therapies can be chosen that are most appropriate to the patient's condition.

AICDs are expensive (costing around £20 000) but effective, a number of trials having shown significant improvements in mortality. They are indicated for patients with a history of:

- ventricular fibrillation or ventricular tachycardia (not due to a transient or reversible cause)
- syncope (where haemodynamically significant ventricular arrhythmias can be induced during electrophysiological studies (EPS) and where drug therapy is ineffective or cannot be used)
- non-sustained ventricular tachycardia in the setting of ischaemic cardiomyopathy where ventricular arrhythmias can be induced during EPS and are not suppressible using Class I anti-arrhythmic agents.

AICDs are usually capable of acting as permanent pacemakers during episodes of bradycardia.

15

AMBULATORY ECG RECORDING

The ECG is a key investigation in patients with palpitations. However, most patients who complain of palpitations only experience them intermittently. One of the limitations of the 12-lead ECG is that, in patients with a history of intermittent palpitations, it is often entirely normal between episodes.

Although a 12-lead ECG recorded while the patient is asymptomatic might indicate the probable nature of the arrhythmia (for instance, the finding of a short PR interval makes atrioventricular re-entry tachycardia a likely diagnosis, whereas a long QT interval makes ventricular tachycardia (VT) more likely), there is no substitute for obtaining an ECG recording **during** an episode of palpitations. There are five ways in which this can be achieved:

- 24-h ambulatory ECG recording
- event recorder
- ECG 'on demand'
- bedside monitoring/telemetry (inpatient)
- implantable loop recorder.

Table 15.1 provides a guide to which modality of investigation is most likely to capture an ECG during an episode of palpitations, depending upon the frequency of the patient's symptoms.

Table 15.1 Probability of capturing an episode of palpitations

Investigation method	Period between episodes		
	Days	Weeks	Months
24-hour ambulatory ECG recording	+++	+	+
Event recorder	+++	++	+
ECG 'on demand'	+++[a]	+++[a]	+++[a]
Bedside monitoring/telemetry (inpatient)	+++	+	+
Implantable loop recorder	+++	+++	+++

+++ = good; ++ = fair; + = poor.
[a] Only helpful if the patient is able to obtain an ECG during a symptomatic episode.

24-HOUR AMBULATORY ECG RECORDING

The 24-h ambulatory ECG recording (Holter monitor) is one of the most frequently requested investigations in the assessment of patients with palpitations. The recorder is carried by the patient on a strap or belt and records the ECG via a small number of electrodes applied to the skin. The recording may be made onto a cassette tape or digitally in a solid-state device. After the device is returned, the recording is analysed using appropriate software, looking for any rhythm disturbance.

One of the main drawbacks of the 24-h ambulatory ECG recorder is its short duration. Although recordings can take place over 48 h or even longer, the recording is usually only of value if the patient happens to experience an episode of palpitations while wearing it. If a patient's symptoms are occurring on a daily basis, or two or three times a week, there is a reasonable probability of capturing an ECG during a symptomatic episode. With less frequent symptoms, the 24-h ambulatory ECG recording is much less likely to be informative.

Patients with palpitations are often reassured that their 24-h ECG recording was normal and no further investigations are arranged. This kind of false reassurance is a cause of great concern, as even patients with life-threatening arrhythmias may well have entirely normal ECG recordings between events. The key question to ask any patient about their 24-h ECG recording is: 'Did you experience your typical symptoms during the recording?' If the answer is 'No', the recording should be regarded as non-diagnostic and further investigation may need to be arranged.

Patients should always keep a symptom diary during the recording to help their recollection of events, and should be asked to note the exact time that any events occurred. During analysis of the recording, particular attention must be paid to those periods of the recording during which symptoms occurred, to allow accurate correlation between the symptoms experienced by the patient and their cardiac rhythm at the time.

EVENT RECORDER

Event recorders are usually carried by the patient for longer periods than 24-h or 48-h ambulatory ECG recorders, the main difference being that they are used only to record the ECG during symptomatic episodes rather than continuously. In order to use an event recorder, the patient must be able to activate the device whenever symptoms occur – a recording is then obtained for a pre-determined duration (often around 30 s). With some devices, the patient can then transmit the recording back to the hospital by telephone for an immediate analysis of the cardiac rhythm.

There are two main types of event recorder: those that are continuously attached to the patient via ECG electrodes, and those that are only applied to the chest during an episode of palpitations. The former type is really just an extension of 24-h ambulatory ECG recording, the main difference being that the ECG is not recorded continuously, but instead is only recorded for a short period whenever the patient activates the device. Practical considerations (such as washing and skin irritation from the electrodes) mean that patients can usually only wear this type of event recorder for 7 days. The latter type is usually a small device that can be carried in the patient's pocket for as long as required. The device is held against the skin (usually over the anterior chest wall) and activated whenever symptoms occur.

Patients with relatively infrequent symptoms (occurring, for instance, on a weekly rather than a daily basis) can carry an event recorder in the hope of obtaining an ECG recording during a typical symptomatic episode. If the symptoms are less frequent (e.g. occurring every few months), an event recorder is unlikely to be helpful.

ECG 'ON DEMAND'

In principle, one of the most effective ways to obtain an ECG recording during an episode of palpitations is to ask the patient to attend for an urgent ECG as soon as they notice the onset of symptoms. Practically, however, this approach poses a number of difficulties.

- The symptoms may not last long enough to give the patient time to reach a facility with an ECG machine.
- The patient may not have transport available and it may be inadvisable for them to drive or to travel unaccompanied while symptomatic.
- The patient may be asked to wait in line for an ECG when they arrive, by which time their symptoms may have resolved.

Nonetheless, this can be a rewarding approach, particularly if a patient's symptoms are relatively mild and infrequent (e.g. only occurring every few weeks or months) but last for long enough for them to reach a facility with an ECG machine. The patient should be given a form or letter (see the box below) and advised to take it to their nearest primary care physician or hospital emergency room (or ECG department) when they develop symptoms. The letter should be on official notepaper and request that whoever sees the patient should perform a 12-lead ECG **as soon as possible** if the patient presents with symptoms. The letter should also give an address to which a copy of the ECG should be sent **and,** in case the ECG goes astray, should ask that the patient also be given a copy to keep. The patient should then bring any ECGs recorded in this way to their next consultation.

Suggested letter format for ECG 'on demand'

To Whom It May Concern

Re: [*insert patient's details here*]

The above-named patient is currently undergoing investigation for palpitations. They have been instructed to try to obtain a 12-lead ECG if they experience a symptomatic episode.

If the patient presents to you with palpitations, please would you obtain a good-quality 12-lead ECG recording **as rapidly as possible** (before the symptoms resolve). Please note on the ECG recording whether the patient's symptoms were still present at the time of the recording.

I would be grateful if you would send a copy of the ECG to [*insert physician's details here*]. Please also give a copy to the patient to bring to their next consultation.

Thank you.

[*Insert name and signature here*]

BEDSIDE MONITORING/TELEMETRY (INPATIENT)

If the palpitations are frequent (e.g. daily) and sufficiently troublesome to merit an urgent diagnosis, one option that is likely to yield a diagnosis is to admit the patient to hospital and use a bedside cardiac monitor (or telemetry). The patient should be instructed to inform the nursing staff immediately whenever they experience palpitations so that the monitor can be checked and a recording obtained. Many bedside ECG monitors now incorporate diagnostic software that is sophisticated enough to detect most (but not all) significant arrhythmias, sound an alarm and store (or print out) a rhythm strip.

This approach can be effective at obtaining a diagnosis, but its limitations are that it can be expensive, it can be inconvenient for patients and it takes patients out of their 'everyday' environment and activities, which might affect the frequency of their symptoms.

IMPLANTABLE LOOP RECORDER

The patient who experiences severe but infrequent symptoms, such as unheralded syncope occurring once every few months, presents one of the most challenging problems. In this case the urgent need to identify a potentially dangerous rhythm disturbance (such as VT or intermittent third-degree atrioventricular block) is made more difficult by its infrequent occurrence. Even an event recorder is a rather hit-and-miss method of capturing symptomatic episodes and, if the patient loses consciousness, they may not be able to activate a recorder until after the rhythm disturbance has resolved and they have regained consciousness.

An implantable loop recorder (such as Medtronic's Reveal Plus device) provides a useful means of attempting to capture an ECG during one of these infrequent episodes. The device is small (and has no attached leads) and is implanted subcutaneously in a similar position to a permanent pacemaker. It contains a battery (which lasts approximately 14 months) and a digital recorder that monitors the ECG and records a rhythm strip. The recorder works on a loop principle, so that the earliest rhythm recording is continuously overwritten by the latest on a continuous 'rolling' basis. At any one time around 20 min of the current cardiac rhythm are stored in the device's memory, although the amount of storage available varies according to the device and its settings.

If an event occurs, the recording loop can be 'frozen' by the patient using an activation device that is held against the recorder – this recording can then be downloaded at a later date by the centre where the unit was implanted. The latest devices also contain diagnostic software that can be programmed to identify and store even asymptomatic rhythm disturbances. There is sufficient memory in the device to record several loops before a download is necessary.

The implantable loop recorder represents a useful way to record the ECG in those patients whose symptoms are infrequent but nonetheless worrying. Its usefulness has to be weighed against the need for an invasive procedure (with the associated risks of scarring and infection) and the cost of the device, although the cost is somewhat offset by the reduced need for multiple non-invasive ambulatory recordings.

16

EXERCISE ECG TESTING

The exercise ECG can be a valuable tool for the assessment of patients with ischaemic heart disease and exercise-related arrhythmias. However, failure to interpret exercise ECGs correctly limits their usefulness.

In this chapter, we will help you to answer the following questions:

- What are the indications for an exercise ECG?
- What are the risks of an exercise ECG?
- How do I perform an exercise ECG?
- When do I stop an exercise ECG?
- How do I interpret an exercise ECG?

WHAT ARE THE INDICATIONS FOR AN EXERCISE ECG?

Exercise ECG testing can be useful in:

- diagnosing chest pain
- risk stratification in stable angina
- risk stratification after myocardial infarction
- assessing exercise-induced arrhythmias
- assessing the need for a permanent pacemaker
- assessing exercise tolerance
- assessing response to treatment.

Exercise ECG testing should always be undertaken with a specific question in mind, and an appreciation of its limitations. In particular, it should only be performed if the information you are likely to gain outweighs the potential (albeit small) risks.

WHAT ARE THE RISKS OF AN EXERCISE ECG?

As with all procedures, exercise ECG testing carries risks:

- a morbidity of 2.4 in 10 000
- a mortality of 1 in 10 000 (within 1 week of testing).

To minimize the risks, always take a patient history and perform an examination to check for **absolute** contraindications to exercise ECG testing (Table 16.1).

Table 16.1 Absolute contraindications to an exercise ECG

- Recent myocardial infarction (within 7 days)
- Unstable angina (rest pain within previous 48 h)
- Severe aortic stenosis or hypertrophic obstructive cardiomyopathy
- Acute myocarditis
- Acute pericarditis
- Uncontrolled hypertension
  - systolic BP > 250 mmHg
  - diastolic BP > 120 mmHg
- Uncontrolled heart failure
- Recent thromboembolic episode (pulmonary or systemic)
- Acute febrile illness

In addition, there are several **relative** contraindications to exercise testing, in the presence of which the test should only be performed with a full awareness of the increased risks involved and under close medical supervision (Table 16.2).

HOW DO I PERFORM AN EXERCISE ECG?

Unless the exercise test is being performed to assess the effectiveness of therapy, patients should be advised to tail off any existing anti-anginal treatment over the 3 days before

Table 16.2 Relative contraindications to an exercise ECG

- Recent myocardial infarction (within 7 days to 1 month)[a]
- Known **severe** coronary artery disease
- Known serious risk of arrhythmia
- Mild or moderate aortic stenosis or hypertrophic obstructive cardiomyopathy
- Pulmonary hypertension
- Significant left ventricular dysfunction
- Aneurysm (ventricular or aortic)
- Highly abnormal resting ECG[b]
  - left or right bundle branch block
  - digoxin effect
- Frail patients

[a] A submaximal exercise test should be used.
[b] An exercise thallium scan can be considered instead.

the test. They can use sublingual glyceryl trinitrate until 1 h before the test.

On the day of the test, ensure that two people – trained in cardiopulmonary resuscitation (CPR) – are present for supervision and that all the necessary drugs and equipment for CPR are available.

After explaining the test to the patient and checking for contraindications (see previous section), decide which exercise protocol to use. There are many different protocols available, but the two most commonly used are:

- the Bruce protocol
- the modified Bruce protocol.

The modified Bruce protocol begins with a lighter workload than the Bruce protocol, and is particularly suitable for frail patients or those being assessed after a recent myocardial infarction (Fig. 16.1).

After reviewing the patient's resting ECG and checking their blood pressure, they can commence exercise. Monitor their symptoms and ECG throughout, and check their blood pressure every 3 min. Reasons for stopping the test are discussed below.

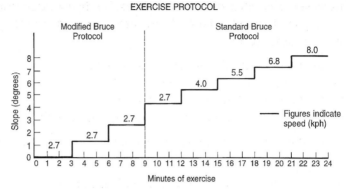

Fig. 16.1 The Bruce and modified Bruce protocols

Protocol	Modified Bruce			Standard Bruce				
Stage	01	02	03	1	2	3	4	5
Speed (kph)	2.7	2.7	2.7	2.7	4.0	5.5	6.8	8.0
Slope (degrees)	0	1.3	2.6	4.3	5.4	6.3	7.2	8.1

After the completion of exercise, continue to monitor the patient's ECG and blood pressure until any symptoms or ECG changes have fully resolved.

What is a MET?

The workload at each level of an exercise protocol can be expressed in terms of metabolic equivalents (or METs). One MET, the rate of oxygen consumption by a normal person at rest, is 3.5 mL/kg per min. To perform the activities of daily living requires 5 METs.

WHEN DO I STOP AN EXERCISE ECG?

One indicator of a good prognosis is the ability to achieve a target heart rate with no symptoms or significant ECG changes. The target heart rate is calculated thus:

Target heart rate = 220 − patient's age (in years)

However, a number of events may require the exercise test to be stopped before the target heart rate is reached. The test *must* be stopped if:

- the patient asks for the test to be stopped
- the systolic blood pressure falls by >20 mmHg
- the heart rate falls by >10 beats/min
- sustained ventricular or supraventricular arrhythmias occur.

In addition, you should consider stopping the test if the patient develops:

- >2 mm ST segment depression and chest pain
- >3 mm asymptomatic ST segment depression
- conduction disturbance and chest pain
- non-sustained ventricular tachycardia
- dizziness
- marked or disproportionate breathlessness
- severe fatigue or exhaustion.

HOW DO I INTERPRET AN EXERCISE ECG?

If the exercise ECG was done to induce an exercise-related arrhythmia, it should be fairly clear whether the test has succeeded in doing so. The interpretation of arrhythmias is the subject of the earlier chapters in this book. Repeating the exercise test once the patient has been established on treatment can be helpful in assessing its efficacy.

Exercise ECGs performed for ischaemic heart disease are often poorly interpreted, and part of the reason for this is a failure to appreciate their limitations. Exercise ECG testing is *not* a 'gold-standard' test for ischaemic heart disease, and so you should be careful about reporting tests in 'black or white' terms such as 'positive' or 'negative'. It may be more useful instead to estimate the probability that a patient has coronary artery disease (see below).

The most common indicator of coronary artery disease upon exercise is the development of ST segment depression, and the greater the depression, the higher the probability of coronary artery disease. However, care must be taken when measuring ST segment depression during exercise, as depression of the **J point** (the junction of the S wave and ST segment) is normal. The ST segment upslopes sharply after the J point, and returns to the baseline within 60 ms (1.5 small squares). You must therefore measure ST segment depression **80 ms (2 small squares) beyond the J point** (Fig. 16.2).

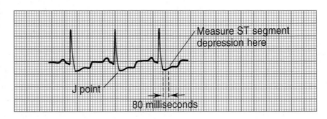

Fig. 16.2 The J point

Key points: ● the J point is the junction of the S wave and ST segment

● measure ST segment depression 80 ms after the J point

ST segment depression is not the only significant result, however. T wave inversion may develop during exercise, as may bundle branch block, although these can occur without significant coronary artery disease. A fall in systolic blood pressure often indicates severe coronary artery disease.

The ECGs in Fig. 16.3 were recorded in a patient with three-vessel coronary artery disease, and show the ST segment changes before, during and after exercise.

The probability of a patient having coronary artery disease depends upon:

● gender (fewer false positives in men)
● age (fewer false positives in older patients)
● degree of ST segment depression
● accompanying symptoms.

Table 16.3 allows you to estimate a patient's probability of coronary artery disease based upon these parameters.

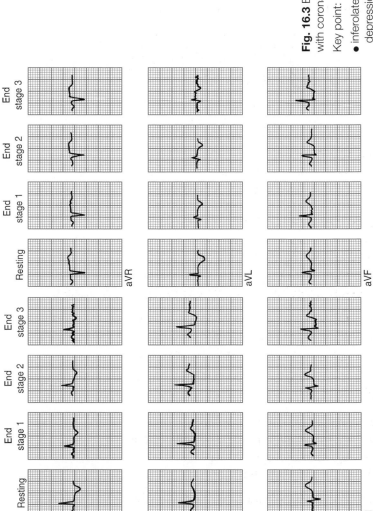

Fig. 16.3 Exercise test in a patient with coronary artery disease

Key point:

- inferolateral ST segment depression during exercise

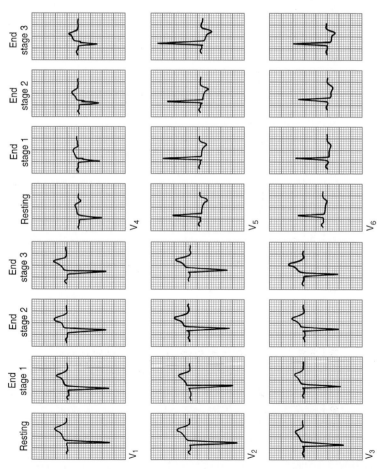

Fig. 16.3 (continued)

Table **16.3** Probability (%) of coronary artery disease according to age, sex and exercise test findings

Age (years)	ST segment depression (mm)	Male patients				Female patients			
		Symptoms				Symptoms			
		None	Non-anginal chest pain	Atypical angina	Typical angina	None	Non-anginal chest pain	Atypical angina	Typical angina
30–39	0–0.5	<1	1	6	25	<1	<1	1	7
	0.5–1.0	2	5	21	68	<1	1	4	24
	1.0–1.5	4	10	38	83	1	2	9	42
	1.5–2.0	8	19	55	91	1	3	16	59
	2.0–2.5	18	38	76	96	3	8	33	79
	>2.5	43	68	92	99	11	24	63	93
40–49	0–0.5	1	4	16	61	<1	1	3	22
	0.5–1.0	5	13	44	86	1	3	12	53
	1.0–1.5	11	26	64	94	2	6	25	72
	1.5–2.0	20	41	78	97	4	11	39	84
	2.0–2.5	39	65	91	99	10	24	63	93
	>2.5	69	87	97	>99	28	53	86	98

(continued)

Table 16.3 (continued)

Age (years)	ST segment depression (mm)	Male patients Symptoms				Female patients Symptoms			
		None	Non-anginal chest pain	Atypical angina	Typical angina	None	Non-anginal chest pain	Atypical angina	Typical angina
50–59	0–0.5	2	6	25	73	1	2	10	47
	0.5–1.0	9	20	57	91	3	8	31	78
	1.0–1.5	19	37	75	96	7	16	50	89
	1.5–2.0	31	53	86	98	12	28	67	94
	2.0–2.5	54	75	94	99	27	50	84	98
	>2.5	81	91	98	>99	56	78	95	99
60–69	0–0.5	3	8	32	79	2	5	21	69
	0.5–1.0	11	26	65	94	7	17	52	90
	1.0–1.5	23	45	81	97	15	33	72	95
	1.5–2.0	37	62	90	99	25	49	83	98
	2.0–2.5	61	81	96	>99	47	72	93	99
	>2.5	85	94	99	>99	76	90	98	>99

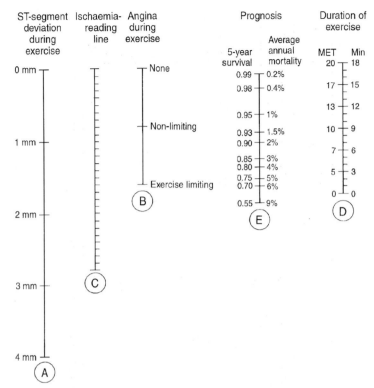

Fig. 16.4 Nomogram for predicting prognosis following exercise testing (Adapted from Mark D.B. et al. 1991. *N Engl J Med* **325**, 849–53. Copyright 1996, Massachusetts Medical Society. All rights reserved.)

How to use:

- mark on line A the maximum ST segment deviation seen during exercise
- mark on line B the degree of angina during exercise
- join the marks on lines A and B with a straight line
- mark the point where this line crosses line C (the 'ischaemia-reading line')
- mark on line D the duration of exercise (Bruce protocol) or METs achieved
- join the marks on lines C and D with a straight line
- where this line crosses line E, read off the patient's predicted mortality

The results of exercise ECG testing also allow for risk stratification by using a nomogram, such as the one in Fig. 16.4, to predict mortality.

17

CARDIOPULMONARY RESUSCITATION

Many cardiac arrests are poorly managed because of disorganization of the cardiac arrest team and a lack of knowledge about recommended procedures by its members. In particular, arrhythmias are frequently incorrectly diagnosed and treated. The rapid identification and treatment of arrhythmias are a cornerstone of successful cardiopulmonary resuscitation (CPR), and for this reason we have included this section on CPR to help you answer the following questions:

- What should I do if a patient collapses?
- How do I perform basic life support (BLS)?
- How do I perform advanced life support?
- How do I diagnose the arrhythmias?
- When – and how – should I use the defibrillator?
- IIow do I treat ventricular fibrillation (VF) and pulseless ventricular tachycardia (VT)?
- How do I treat non-VF/VT rhythms?
- How do I manage peri-arrest arrhythmias?
- How should I direct others during the arrest?
- What should I do after the arrest?

The guidelines in this chapter are based upon the Guidelines of the European Resuscitation Council (2000). If you would like to learn more about Advanced Life Support, there is no substitute for attending a formal training course. In the United Kingdom such courses are coordinated by the Resuscitation Council (UK) and contact details can be found in the 'Further reading' section at the end of this book.

Current teaching in CPR emphasizes the chain of survival – four interventions that contribute to a successful outcome. These are:

- early access to help (from emergency services or a cardiac arrest team)
- early BLS to buy time
- early defibrillation (where appropriate)
- early advanced life support to stabilize the patient.

All four links in the chain must be strong in order to maximize the chances of a successful outcome. All four elements of the chain of survival are covered in this chapter.

WHAT SHOULD I DO IF A PATIENT COLLAPSES?

The concept of BLS assumes that no special equipment is initially available, as might be the case if someone collapses in the street. However, if you are a healthcare professional, it is much more likely that you will attend patients who have collapsed in a healthcare environment, and some modification of the standard BLS protocols is appropriate. This section assumes that the BLS is taking place in a healthcare environment unless otherwise stated.

If you witness a patient collapse or find a patient apparently unresponsive, you should immediately shout for help and then assess whether the patient is responsive by gently shaking them by the shoulders and asking loudly, 'Are you all right?'. If help arrives quickly, the following steps can be undertaken simultaneously.

If the patient is unresponsive, check whether they are breathing (10 s) while simultaneously checking for the carotid pulse (10 s) – see below for more information about doing this. If the patient is pulseless and/or not breathing, you will need to call the cardiac arrest team. One person should commence BLS while another goes to call the cardiac arrest team and collect the defibrillator and resuscitation equipment. If you are the only person present, you should go to obtain help **before** commencing BLS.

If you are attending a casualty outside the healthcare setting, the decision about when to go for help depends upon how many rescuers are present. If there are two or more rescuers, one should go for help as soon as it is clear that the casualty is not breathing. The remaining rescuer should undertake BLS. If you are alone, the decision about when to go for help will depend upon the circumstances and in particular the availability of emergency medical services. If it is probable that the casualty is unconscious because of a breathing problem (as opposed to a heart problem), as is likely in cases of trauma, drowning, drug or alcohol intoxication, or in infants and children, it is advisable to perform 1 min of BLS before going to find help.

HOW DO I PERFORM BASIC LIFE SUPPORT?

Remember the ABC of BLS:

- Airway
- Breathing
- Circulation.

To open the airway, loosen any clothing around the patient's neck and open their mouth. Remove obstructions such as food or loose dentures, but leave well-fitting dentures in place. Tilt the head backward with one hand on the forehead and, using two fingers of the other hand, lift the chin in order to lift the tongue from the back of the throat.

Now assess the patient's breathing by listening at the mouth for breath sounds and feeling for exhaled air on your cheek. Watch the chest for any sign of movement. Continue to observe for 10 s before proceeding.

If the patient is breathing, roll them into the recovery position (unless this may lead to further injury) to lessen the risk of airway obstruction or aspiration. Obtain further assistance, ideally sending someone else to obtain help if possible.

If the patient is not breathing, send someone for help immediately; if you are alone, quickly run for help before giving two rescue breaths. With the patient lying supine, pinch the nose and open the mouth slightly (while tilting the head and lifting the chin). Seal your lips around the patient's mouth and exhale for about 2 s, ensuring that their chest rises. Now take your mouth away, watching that the patient's chest falls. Take another breath, seal your lips around the patient's mouth and exhale, watching again to ensure that the chest rises.

If you are confident in doing so, now palpate the carotid pulse (or do so simultaneously while assessing for signs of breathing). If signs of a circulation are present but the patient is not breathing, expired air respiration should continue at a rate of 10 breaths/min. If the carotid pulse disappears, or if it was absent to begin with, full BLS is required.

Assessing the carotid pulse

For layperson BLS, assessment of the carotid pulse no longer forms part of the standard protocol unless the rescuer is skilled in doing it. This is because assessment of the carotid pulse is time consuming and the decision about the presence or absence of the pulse is, in unskilled hands, often wrong.
If you are unsure about the presence of a circulation, chest compression should be performed.

With the patient lying on a firm surface, open the airway and commence chest compression. Placing the heel of one hand in the middle of the lower half of the patient's sternum (two finger-breadths above the xiphisternum), place the heel of your other hand over the first, interlocking your fingers. Lean directly over the patient with straight arms and press vertically downward, so that the sternum is depressed by 4–5 cm.

Keeping your hands in position, release the pressure and repeat the chest compression at a rate of 100 compressions/min. The time taken for each chest compression should equal the time taken to release the pressure. Follow every 15 chest compressions with two ventilations. A cerebral blood flow of at least 20 per cent of normal needs to be maintained for a full neurological recovery.

With two rescuers, either one rescuer can alternately perform both chest compressions and expired air respiration (at a ratio of 15:2), or (preferably) one rescuer can perform chest compressions while the other performs expired air respiration (again at a ratio of 15:2). If the patient has been successfully intubated, there is no need to stop chest compressions while ventilating the patient.

HOW DO I PERFORM ADVANCED LIFE SUPPORT?

Advanced life support commences as soon as you have access to a defibrillator and suitable drugs. When a full cardiac arrest team is present in hospital, specific tasks can be assigned to individuals (see page 261).

Lose no time in attaching a cardiac monitor to the patient (alternatively, you can monitor the ECG through the defibrillator paddles) and assessing the cardiac rhythm to make a diagnosis. You must make sure that CPR continues until you have decided what the heart rhythm is. Nominate specific individuals to take over BLS at regular intervals, as resuscitation can be very tiring.

HOW DO I DIAGNOSE THE ARRHYTHMIAS?

Remember: time is of the essence. Rapid and correct identification and treatment of cardiac rhythm abnormalities are central to the delivery of effective advanced life support.

You must be able to recognize with confidence each of the four arrhythmias that occur in cardiac arrest:

- VF
- pulseless VT
- asystole
- pulseless electrical activity (PEA).

In addition, you should know how to manage three arrhythmias (discussed later in this chapter) that may appear during or shortly after cardiac arrest:

- bradycardia
- narrow-complex tachycardia
- broad-complex tachycardia.

Ventricular fibrillation

VF is the commonest initial arrhythmia causing cardiac arrest and appears as a chaotic rhythm on the ECG (Fig. 17.1). If the monitor is faulty, or the gain turned too low, it can be mistaken for asystole.

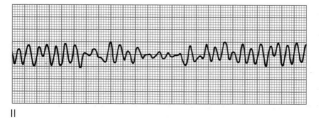

Fig. 17.1
Ventricular fibrillation

Key point:

- chaotic ventricular activity

II

Pulseless ventricular tachycardia

VT appears as a broad-complex rapid cardiac rhythm (Fig. 17.2), and can cause haemodynamic collapse (hence 'pulseless').

Asystole

Asystole implies there is no spontaneous electrical cardiac activity, and thus the ECG shows no QRS complexes (Fig. 17.3).

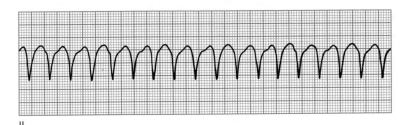

II

Fig. 17.2 Ventricular tachycardia

Key point: ● broad-complex tachycardia

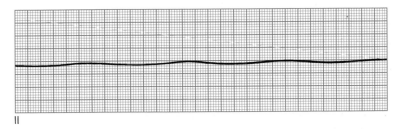

II

Fig. 17.3 Asystole

Key point: ● no spontaneous electrical activity

P waves may persist for a short time after the onset of ventricular asystole (and are an indicator that the patient may respond to ventricular pacing). Beware of mistaking 'fine VF', or VF with a low gain setting on the monitor, for asystole. If there is any doubt as to whether the rhythm is fine VF or asystole, initial treatment should begin with defibrillation. Beware, too, of diagnosing asystole when you see a completely flat line on the monitor – there is usually some baseline drift in asystole and the line is seldom completely flat. A perfectly flat line is more likely to be due to a faulty electrode or connection.

Pulseless electrical activity

PEA is sometimes called electromechanical dissociation, and occurs when the heart continues to work electrically (the ECG continues to show QRS complexes, Fig. 17.4), but fails to provide a circulation. Reasons for this include massive pulmonary embolism (obstructing blood flow), large myocardial infarction (causing mechanical 'weakness' of the heart muscle) and severe haemorrhage (loss of circulating volume).

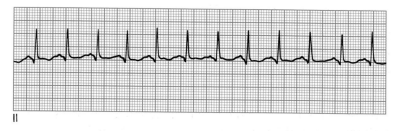

II

Fig. 17.4 Pulseless electrical activity

Key point: ● QRS complexes (in the absence of a cardiac output)

Cardiac rhythms in PEA

It is important to remember that PEA can exist in conjunction with **any** of the cardiac rhythms that would normally sustain a circulation, not just sinus rhythm.

Patients with atrial fibrillation or with an atrioventricular (AV) re-entry tachycardia, for instance, should normally have a pulse – in the absence of a pulse, they have PEA.

Having confidently diagnosed the rhythm disorder, move on quickly to provide the appropriate treatment.

WHEN – AND HOW – SHOULD I USE THE DEFIBRILLATOR?

Defibrillation is used during a cardiac arrest to convert the heart from an abnormal rhythm to sinus rhythm (or, at least, to a rhythm that restores a cardiac output). Hence, you must use the defibrillator when you have diagnosed:

- VF
- pulseless VT.

In addition, you should defibrillate the patient if you think they are in asystole but cannot be **entirely** confident that it isn't small complex ('fine') VF.

However, there is no point in defibrillating a patient if you are **confident** that they are in asystole. Defibrillation just changes one rhythm to another – it will not restart the heart when there is no initial rhythm.

There is also no point in defibrillating pulseless electrical activity. By definition, the heart is working normally electrically – you have to find a mechanical reason for the lack of a cardiac output.

Ensure you are familiar with the defibrillators used in your workplace, as you cannot afford to waste time should you need to use one. Many units now use biphasic (rather than monophasic) defibrillators – these lower the defibrillation threshold and so lower shock energies are required.

Apply electrode jelly or preferably gel pads to the skin below the paddles, but do not spread jelly between the paddles as this can cause a 'short-circuit'. Note also that some gel pads need replacing between shocks.

After warning everyone to stand clear, perform a 'visual sweep' to check that:

- everyone (including yourself!) is clear of the patient and the bed
- no-one is touching drip stands connected to the patient
- high-flow oxygen is not passing across the zone of defibrillation
- all transdermal medication patches have been removed from the patient (risk of burns if they have a metal backing)

● the paddles are at least 15 cm from any permanent pacemaker box.

Finally, look one last time at the monitor to check the rhythm hasn't changed and, if appropriate, proceed to deliver the direct current (DC) shocks (as described in the appropriate protocol) without delay.

Precordial thump

A precordial thump may deliver sufficient energy to restore an effective rhythm in 2 per cent of cases of VF and in up to 40 per cent of cases of VT. However, it must be delivered rapidly, within 30 s of the start of the arrhythmia. The precordial thump should be considered if an arrest is witnessed or monitored and if a defibrillator is not immediately to hand. It is administered with a single sharp blow over the patient's sternum using a closed fist.

HOW DO I TREAT VF AND PULSELESS VT?

Both arrhythmias are treated identically (Fig. 17.5). Electrical defibrillation must be provided as quickly as possible, as described in the previous section. Start with three DC shocks in rapid succession, at energies of 200 J, 200 J and then 360 J (for monophasic systems – optimal energy levels for biphasic systems have yet to be determined). Pause only briefly between shocks to reassess the patient's rhythm (and pulse if there is a change in rhythm) and to recharge the defibrillator. If all three shocks can be delivered in less than 60 s, it is not necessary to resume BLS between each shock.

Continue BLS for 1 min and then reassess the cardiac rhythm and pulse. During CPR, establish intravenous access using either the external jugular vein or a large antecubital vein. If a peripheral vein is used, flush it with 20 mL of isotonic saline after administering each drug. The patient should be intubated at this point.

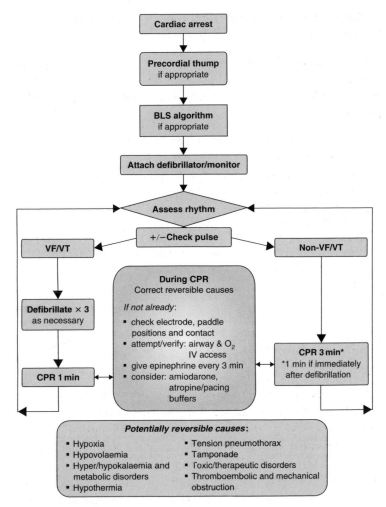

Fig. 17.5 The advanced life support (ALS) universal algorithm for the management of cardiac arrest in adults

Source: *ALS Provider Manual*, 4th edition. Reproduced with the kind permission of the Resuscitation Council (UK).

Do not delay BLS for more than 15 s when attempting intravenous access and intubation. If the attempts fail, wait until after the next set of DC shocks before trying again. Whether the attempts succeed or not, recommence chest compression and ventilation at a ratio of 15:2 for 1 min. Once the patient has been successfully intubated, chest compression and ventilation can take place concurrently rather than sequentially. Remember to give epinephrine (adrenaline) 1 mg intravenously (or 2–3 mg, diluted to at least 10 mL with sterile water, via the endotracheal tube and followed by five ventilations) every 3 min during the cardiac arrest to help maintain myocardial and cerebral perfusion pressures.

 DRUG POINT

Epinephrine acts as a peripheral vasoconstrictor, reducing blood flow to the skin and skeletal muscle and thereby increasing cerebral and myocardial blood flow.

Continue BLS for 1 min and assess the cardiac rhythm and pulse. If a satisfactory rhythm has still not been restored, deliver three more DC shocks, each at an energy of 360 J. The 'loop' should be repeated until either a perfusing rhythm is restored or it is decided that continued CPR would be inappropriate. If a perfusing rhythm is restored but then VF/pulseless VT recurs, the next set of shocks should revert back to 200 J, 200 J and then 360 J thereafter.

If the patient remains in VF, try changing the paddle positions to anteroposterior or changing the defibrillator itself. After the third set of shocks, consider drugs such as amiodarone (or lidocaine (lignocaine) if amiodarone is unavailable), magnesium (if hypomagnesaemia is suspected), and bicarbonate (if pH < 7.1 and/or the cardiac arrest is associated with a tricyclic overdose or hyperkalaemia). However, evidence of benefit is lacking.

HOW DO I TREAT NON-VF/VT RHYTHMS?

Asystole and PEA are associated with relatively poor outcomes unless a treatable cause can be identified. The potentially reversible causes of cardiac arrest are listed in Table 17.1 and are commonly known as the 'four Hs and four Ts'.

Table 17.1 Potentially reversible causes of cardiac arrest

- Hypoxia
- Hypovolaemia
- Hypothermia
- Hypokalaemia and hyperkalaemia (and other metabolic disorders)
- Tension pneumothorax
- Thromboembolism (and other mechanical obstruction)
- Tamponade
- Toxic and therapeutic disorders

Asystole

Always beware of incorrectly diagnosing VF as asystole. This can occur as a result of misinterpretation, faulty equipment or too low a gain setting on the monitor. **If in any doubt**, administer three DC shocks at energies of 200 J, 200 J and 360 J to avoid missing a potentially reversible arrhythmia.

Following the shocks (or if you can confidently diagnose asystole from the outset), start BLS, intubate the patient and obtain intravenous access. Administer epinephrine 1 mg intravenously and maintain BLS for 3 min. Consider giving atropine 3 mg intravenously (or 6 mg in a volume of 10–20 mL via the endotracheal tube).

 DRUG POINT

Atropine acts by reducing vagal (parasympathetic) nerve activity on the heart and thereby increases the heart rate, although its value in asystole has not been proven.

If P waves or slow ventricular activity are present, consider pacing (Chapter 14). If asystole persists, repeat the loop, maintaining BLS and giving further doses of epinephrine every 3 min. High-dose epinephrine is no longer recommended.

If the rhythm changes to VF/pulseless VT, reassess the pulse and, as appropriate, switch to the VF/pulseless VT algorithm.

Pulseless electrical activity

If you diagnose PEA, always look hard for an underlying remediable cause (see Table 17.1). Support the patient in the same way as for asystole with CPR and give epinephrine 1 mg intravenously every 3 min. If PEA is associated with bradycardia, atropine 3 mg intravenously can be given.

HOW DO I MANAGE PERI-ARREST ARRHYTHMIAS?

You must be able to recognize and be prepared to treat promptly any arrhythmia that develops during or shortly after cardiac arrest. Always be alert to adverse signs that will help determine the response to the arrhythmia (Table 17.2).

Table 17.2 Adverse clinical signs during arrhythmias

- Systolic blood pressure <90 mmHg
- Low cardiac output (poor perfusion, impaired conscious level)
- Excessive tachycardia (>200/min for narrow-complex tachycardia, >150/min for broad-complex tachycardia)
- Excessive bradycardia (<40/min)
- Heart failure (pulmonary or peripheral congestion)
- Myocardial ischaemia (chest pain or ST segment changes)

Bradycardia

You should quickly assess the patient's ECG and clinical condition, as these will help you decide the likelihood of their condition deteriorating. A ventricular rate <40/min is regarded as excessively slow, although patients may be acutely unwell even at higher rates if they have poor underlying cardiac function. The presence of adverse clinical signs is an indication for atropine. Atropine 500 mcg intravenously will usually increase the heart rate, but several doses may be needed up to a maximum total of 3 mg.

Table 17.3 Predictors of asystole

- Recent asystole
- Mobitz type II AV block
- Third-degree AV block with broad QRS complexes
- Ventricular pauses >3.0 s

If there is a risk of asystole (Table 17.3), pacing is likely to be needed. Seek expert advice, as temporary pacing may be necessary. As a temporary measure, atropine, external pacing or an infusion of intravenous epinephrine may be used.

 SEEK HELP

Expert help may be needed for patients with a peri-arrest bradycardia where there is a risk of asystole or which does not respond to atropine.

Narrow-complex tachycardia

If the narrow-complex tachycardia is due to **atrial fibrillation**, the management depends upon the clinical findings. In high-risk patients (ventricular rate >150/min with adverse clinical findings) expert help should be sought with a view to urgent DC cardioversion. In low-risk patients (ventricular rate <100/min with mild or no adverse clinical findings), anticoagulation and rate control (if required) may be the only immediate steps necessary. The situation is more complex for those patients who belong to an intermediate group. Anticoagulation should always be considered, but the decision about rate control and/or DC cardioversion should be taken with the benefit of expert advice.

If the narrow-complex tachycardia is due to a **re-entry tachycardia** – such as AV re-entry tachycardia or AV nodal re-entry tachycardia – and the patient is pulseless (which is rare and usually only seen with a rate of >250/min),

a synchronized DC shock at a monophasic energy level of 100 J is required. If the patient is not pulseless, after administering oxygen and gaining intravenous access, vagal manoeuvres can be attempted to try to terminate the tachycardia.
If vagal manoeuvres are unsuccessful (or contraindicated), intravenous adenosine can be considered (but with caution in Wolff–Parkinson–White syndrome).

If this is unsuccessful, seek expert help if you have not already done so. In the presence of adverse clinical signs, preparations should be made for DC cardioversion under sedation. With the defibrillator set to *synchronized* mode, give a 100 J shock and reassess the patient. If the arrhythmia persists, try further shocks of 200 J and 360 J. An infusion of amiodarone may improve the chances of successful DC cardioversion to sinus rhythm. In the absence of adverse clinical signs, treatment can be given with esmolol, digoxin, verapamil or amiodarone – all are effective and most hospitals will stock at least two of these drugs. Exceptionally, overdrive pacing may be necessary.

Broad-complex tachycardia

Always feel the carotid or other large artery for a pulse – if you cannot feel one, give a precordial thump and follow the VF/pulseless VT protocol (see Fig. 17.5).

Next, look for evidence of adverse clinical signs. If present, you should get expert help quickly and prepare to sedate the patient for DC cardioversion. With the defibrillator set to *synchronized* mode, give a 100 J shock and reassess the patient. If the arrhythmia persists, try further shocks of 200 J and 360 J. An infusion of intravenous amiodarone can be effective in improving the efficacy of cardioversion if the initial shocks are unsuccessful. If serum levels of potassium are low, these should be corrected and in addition magnesium should be given intravenously. In exceptional cases, alternative anti-arrhythmic drugs (such as lidocaine, procainamide or sotalol) or overdrive pacing may be necessary.

If adverse clinical signs are not present, start treatment at once with an infusion of either amiodarone or lidocaine, correct serum potassium if this is low and give magnesium intravenously. If the arrhythmia persists, arrange to cardiovert the patient and call for expert help.

HOW SHOULD I DIRECT OTHERS DURING THE ARREST?

A poorly trained and inexperienced arrest team will conduct a cardiac arrest in a disorganized manner. It is essential that all members of the team are familiar with basic and advanced life support guidelines and that the most experienced person present takes overall control of the situation.

While diagnosing the arrhythmias and taking decisions accordingly, the team leader must direct others by giving clear instructions to specified individuals. Ideally, there should be one member of the team for each of the following tasks:

● chest compression (swapping with others when tired)
● defibrillation
● ventilating and/or intubating the patient
● obtaining intravenous access
● drawing up the necessary drugs
● keeping a record of events, and counting the seconds out loud whenever CPR is interrupted.

The team leader should also discuss with the rest of the team when further resuscitation appears futile and, if the others are in agreement, terminate resuscitation efforts.

WHAT SHOULD I DO AFTER THE ARREST?

Following a successful resuscitation, the patient will need observation and monitoring, ideally on an intensive or coronary care unit. Particularly important is the management of the patient's airway and breathing, especially if their conscious level is reduced, and artificial ventilation may be needed.

You will need to monitor:

- airway and breathing (including pulse oximetry)
- vital signs (pulse, blood pressure and temperature)
- peripheral perfusion
- cardiac rhythm
- neurological status (including Glasgow Coma Score)
- urine output and fluid balance

in addition to checking:

- arterial blood gases
- blood urea and electrolytes (including K^+, Mg^{2+} and Ca^{2+})
- chest X-ray
- blood glucose
- 12-lead ECG
- full blood count.

These post-arrest investigations can be remembered by the mnemonic ABCDEF (Arterial blood gases; Biochemistry – blood urea and electrolytes; Chest X-ray; Dextrose – blood glucose; ECG – 12-lead ECG; Full blood count).

Finally, do not forget the patient's relatives. Speak to them as soon as possible after the arrest.

FURTHER READING

ECG INTERPRETATION

Bennett DH (2002) *Cardiac Arrhythmias*, 6th edn. Arnold, ISBN 0340807318.

An excellent guide to the diagnosis and treatment of cardiac arrhythmias.

CARDIOLOGY TEXTBOOKS

Desmond J et al. (1998) *Cardiology*, 7th edn. Saunders, ISBN 070202211X.

A useful handbook for cardiovascular medicine.

Grubb NR, Newby DE (2000) *Churchill's Pocketbook of Cardiology*. Churchill Livingstone, ISBN 0443062218.

A detailed and up-to-date pocket-sized handbook of cardiology.

RESUSCITATION GUIDELINES

In the United Kingdom the teaching of Advanced Life Support is co-ordinated nationally by the Resuscitation Council (UK):

5th Floor   Tel: 020 7388 4678
Tavistock House North   Fax: 020 7383 0773
Tavistock Square   Email: enquiries@resus.org.uk
London WC1H 9HR   Website: www.resus.org.uk

HELP WITH THE NEXT EDITION

We would like to know what you would like to see included (or omitted!) in the next edition of *Making Sense of the ECG*. Please write with your comments or suggestions to:

Dr Andrew R. Houghton
Making Sense of the ECG
c/o Hodder Arnold, Health Sciences
338 Euston Road
London NW1 3BH

We will include acknowledgements to all those whose suggestions are used in the next edition.

INDEX